Understanding Health and Well-Being

This textbook provides a comprehensive introduction to the factors that impact physical, mental, and social well-being, offering a broad definition of health and healthcare that moves beyond the biomedical model.

Stressing that health is not merely the absence of disease or infirmity, the book addresses a diverse range of issues that influence individual, community, and population health. There are chapters on the microbiome, physical activity, and lifestyle and behavior, as well as the various social determinants of health, health literacy, and issues around mental health. Defining health as a wicked problem (i.e., one that is contested and endlessly complicated) the book provides an international lens which also includes coverage of global health and the impact of climate change.

Including key concepts, end-of-chapter questions, and further reading, this is the perfect introductory text for students of public health, health studies, or health sciences.

William Montelpare, Professor, Margaret and Wallace McCain Chair in Human Development and Health, University of Prince Edward Island, Canada.

Amanda Hudson, Director of Research, Planning, and Operations with Health PEI, Mental Health and Addictions, and Adjunct Professor, University of Prince Edward Island, Canada.

Understanding Health and Well-Being

A Holistic Approach to Community Health

William Montelpare and Amanda Hudson

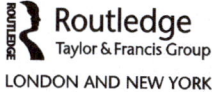

Routledge
Taylor & Francis Group

LONDON AND NEW YORK

Designed cover image: Getty Images

First published 2025
by Routledge
4 Park Square, Milton Park, Abingdon, Oxon OX14 4RN

and by Routledge
605 Third Avenue, New York, NY 10158

Routledge is an imprint of the Taylor & Francis Group, an informa business

British Library Cataloguing-in-Publication Data
A catalogue record for this book is available from the British Library

ISBN: 978-1-032-75604-2 (hbk)
ISBN: 978-1-032-75603-5 (pbk)
ISBN: 978-1-003-47477-7 (ebk)

DOI: 10.4324/9781003474777

Typeset in Sabon
by Apex CoVantage, LLC

Contents

Figures and Tables

Preface

How to Read This Book

Together, we will examine the fundamental concepts of health and healthcare from a comprehensive perspective that has been in a constant state of flux since it was originally presented by the World Health Organization in its 1948 constitutional definition of health as not merely the absence of disease and infirmity, but as a state of physical, mental, and social well-being. From here, we will build on this to include more modern and reflective health concepts from an inclusive, diverse, and equitable perspective.

We realize that the world continues to change daily and that the world in present days is not the world of 1948. Today, there are voices that were silenced or non-existent in 1948, today, there are lines of communication that were not even conceived of in 1948, and yet today, there continue to be challenges both external to the activity of humans and as a result of man's inhumanity to man that inhibit, impair, and restrict the ability for humans to achieve positive health. Throughout our reading, we will explore the importance of lifestyle and of behaviors as essential elements in achieving and maintaining positive states of health while considering potential barriers to attaining health and how the principles of health can be optimized to facilitate health outcomes at the person, community, and population levels.

In striving to realize these objectives, we will identify principles of health based on several influencing factors, including essential stimuli for the development of social, emotional, intellectual, spiritual, and biological health. We will investigate how behavior contributes to one's personal health while recognizing the multifactorial nature of health and the actions one might consider in shaping their personal health.

Understanding current scientific evidence related to health behavior is essential to establishing positive states of health. Throughout this text, advanced concepts and scientific terminology are used, but in many instances, the terms and concepts are explained carefully. Information is cited appropriately and reflects contemporary findings from previously published work. Some specific references reflect the health of Canadian society, but for the most part, the concepts are global and concern individuals from diverse communities.

CHAPTER 1

Essential Background

1.0 Introduction

We begin with the question, "What is health?"

Health is a complex construct with several biases and underlying philosophies. Health is a noun – it is a thing; it can be measured, it can be scaled, it can be achieved, it can be shaped by culture, it can be politicized, and it can be monetized. And yet to achieve a positive state of health, one must overcome specific challenges. These challenges include but are not limited to race, ethnicity, discrimination, acculturation, environment, and socioeconomic status (Pamuk et al., 1998). Both independently and combined, these challenges are complex, and in some circumstances, they become insurmountable obstacles that contribute to the disparities in populations and thereby restrict one's ability to achieve positive states of health.

To be healthy is a dynamic state in which elements of the broad spectrum of social, emotional, physical, spiritual, and economic well-being have been realized.

The constitution of the World Health Organization (WHO), which was initially prepared in 1946, and definitively signed, first by Canada (1946), and later by the United States (1948), defined health as " the state of complete physical, mental, and social well-being and not merely the absence of disease or infirmity."

This early formal definition is important because it advanced the description of an individual's health beyond the mere signs or symptoms of illness. In establishing a concept of health, this statement is a fundamental principle upon which to build knowledge about the multidisciplinary foundation from which health can emerge. Expanding our acceptance that health is not the diametric opposite of illness or infirmity but is based on a broader context enables us to explore health beyond the centeredness of the self.

And yet this definition of health has not been truly understood, nor has it been operationalized. In 1948, the world was a very different place. The world was recovering from the Great Depression and World War II. Jobs were becoming more abundant, and as more folks were working, the price of goods and services increased. Hence, inflation increased. In Canada, the inflation rate was 9% higher in 1948 than in 1947 – this

DOI: 10.4324/9781003474777-1

meant that you had to spend $1.09 for something you only paid $1.00 for in 1947. In the newspaper headlines, Mahatma Gandhi was assassinated in India.

Thirty thousand civilian lives were lost in Taiwanese revolts against Chinese rule (today, Taiwan is considered by China and the U.S.A. as a province of mainland China). The Communists seized power in Czechoslovakia, while the U.S. Congress ratified the Marshall Plan, approving $17 billion in European aid to rebuild Europe following WWII and generate economies for citizens/survivors in Europe.

In healthcare, the world was accepting that the prevention of disease was through vaccination programs. Medicine was becoming mainstream, and by 1954, the Salk polio vaccine had gained favor for widespread application.

During this tremendous societal growth, the notion of health was increasingly medicalized, and defining a healthy individual was primarily associated with an individual's physical state, while mental, economic, and social well-being were relegated to secondary concepts. Unfortunately, the biomedical model, which emerged more than 100 years earlier, was being strengthened as the foundation to defining health. Maintaining a state that was free of disease and free of illness was considered healthy, while providing treatments and medicinal approaches to manage or resolve illness and disease were considered the predominant healthcare practices. Mental health and social well-being were not part of the operational definition of what it meant to achieve a positive state of health. Moreover, recognizing the role of privilege or lack thereof in establishing a state of health was without consideration.

The emerging biomedical model was logical – in the simplest of terms, it could be described as a method to manage the physical signs and reported symptoms of the individual. The biomedical model thus helped to create a cadre of professionals to provide the services needed to ensure that individuals were free of disease and infirmity, regardless of the complexity of causal factors.

The very nature of the biomedical perspective for managing disease and infirmity qualified health to be considered the default to illness. Therefore, if the individual did not show signs or report symptoms of disease or infirmity, then they were not dealing with illness, and hence, they must be healthy.

Yet health is not a dichotomy of health versus illness. Given the original WHO declaration that health is more than merely the absence of disease or infirmity, health cannot be reduced to a dichotomy because health is a multidimensional construct that describes a state of being. Biomedical models cannot describe the multidisciplinary perspective of a state of health because biomedical models are reductionist within the physical dimensions of the person and ignore social and environmental determinants that are part of the Gestalt of health.

Fast-forward to the current day and consider the *limitations* of the biomedical model as a foundation to describing an individual's state of health. If health is more than physical, then the biomedical model is too limited in scope and context to describe an individual's state of health. Establishing determinants of health enables us to create a multivariate model based on metrics that comprehensively define what it means to achieve positive states of health. As noted by Krahn et al., the WHO definition is aspirational, and given that an optimal level of complete health is unachievable, they suggested that health be redefined to include existential well-being in adapting to conditions of life and the environment as part of the definition.

Similar work by van Druten and colleagues concluded that health is undefined and lacks a clear and concise definition that is universally understood. Descriptions of health fail to capture the multifaceted characteristics that underlie the concept of health or what it means to be healthy. Encouragingly, there has been a constant pressure to re-evaluate the definition of health not from a lens of incapacity or physical incapability but from a perspective of capability and potential (Gillon, 1986; Saracci, 1997). To this end, let us examine the factors that determine an individual's state of health. These include the physical, social, and economic environments in which an individual resides. These also include a deeper dive into the precursors to an individual's current state of existence and the role of politics, culture, and social development. The state of an individual's health therefore results from their lived experience, their personal characteristics, and their behaviors within their environment, recognizing that their environment and their capabilities are shaped by multiple factors, many of which are external to the individual's control and which have been entrenched for millennia.

Despite the fact that we may now realize health to encompass concepts beyond the physical dimensions of disease and infirmity (Bradley et al., 2018), much of our world continues to view health as a medicalized enterprise. Unfortunately, medicalizing health constitutes a demand for services of medically trained personnel to provide medical care. The result is that the provision of medical care has erroneously become synonymous with healthcare. For many individuals, this blurring of the lines between medicine – a specific treatment strategy – and health – a gestalt – misinforms the populace and mistakenly strengthens not only the biological model of health but the medicalization of health.

> **Medical care is not synonymous with healthcare – rather, medical care is a part of healthcare.**

Medical care, as in that which is provided most often by frontline physicians, nurses, and other clinicians, includes but is not limited to people that work within the realm of the physical. Medical care is most often a direct treatment or a service to manage an individual's illness or infirmity. Healthcare is a counterpart to medical care and engages the broader notion that includes multiple areas of relevance to an individual's health and includes social, emotional, physical, spiritual, and economic well-being.

1.1 Changing the Narrative on Health and Healthcare

At the 1978 International Conference on Primary Health Care held in Alma-Ata, Kazakhstan, ten declarations were proposed and accepted by conference participants. The declarations included accepting that health is a fundamental human right and that the disparity in health status both between privileged and challenged countries and between advantaged and disadvantaged individuals within a country should be recognized as unacceptable socially, politically, and economically.

If we accept that health is a human right, then we must ensure that all individuals are given the opportunity to attain a level of health that is deemed acceptable. At the Alma-Ata conference, the attendees decided that the modus operandi to achieve a sustained health system for universal health coverage was to strengthen primary healthcare, in turn ensuring a level of health that inclusively addressed people's physical, mental, and social well-being.

Declaration VII was specific in describing primary healthcare as reflecting and evolving from the economic conditions and sociocultural and political characteristics of the country and its communities. This declaration is unambiguous in stating that the principles of primary healthcare are based on the relevant results of social, biomedical, and health services research complemented by the public health experience.

Alma-Ata affirmed that primary healthcare is a cornerstone of a sustainable health system that can provide universal health coverage to all citizens. Moreover, if this is realized, primary healthcare can be the foundation upon which to achieve health-related sustainable development goals.

Importantly, the declarations of Alma-Ata supported that all citizens had not only the right but also the duty to participate in the planning and the delivery of their healthcare. Given that the way forward is for governments to provide opportunities for citizens to achieve adequate health, the onus is on us, individually and collectively, to capitalize on these opportunities and to hold the government accountable to this pledge.

So how do we engage in a process that will ensure effective positive health and healthcare will be achieved for all?

One way is to change our thinking about who is responsible for our health and what being healthy means to us. In fact, once we realize that healthcare is not medical care but actually extends beyond illness, injury, infirmity, and disease treatment in many regards and that healthcare refers to the broader spectrum of social, emotional, physical, spiritual, and economic well-being, then we will begin to take ownership, first of our personal health and then extend that ownership to our shared responsibility for our community, our region, and beyond.

The Greek term *eudaimonia*, refers to well-being or happiness and is an important principle of health. To achieve eudaimonia requires us to optimize health as a dynamic state that engages all elements of the broader spectrum of social, emotional, physical, spiritual, and economic well-being.

In the following chapters, we will explore the different principles of health across the spectrum of health, including the importance of health literacy and how it enables individuals to make informed decisions for themselves. We will also look at health with respect to regional, national, and global policies and practices and the factors which influence decision-making.

1.1.1 Discussion Questions

1   The definition of health is broad and not limited to physical health. How does the expanded definition fit with your sense of health, and how can we relay this information to the general public so that they can gain a better understanding of the gestalt of health?

2   The responsibility for our health lies with us. What are the barriers and challenges to gaining widespread acceptance of this notion? Describe some strategies that can help to advance this concept within the general public.

3   How might we operationalize the World Health Organization's concept of achieving societal well-being, given your definition of health?

References

Bradley, K. L., Goetz, T., and Viswanathan, S. Toward a contemporary definition of health. *Mil Med*. 2018;183(11/12):204.

Gillon, R. On sickness and on health. *Br Med J (Clin Res Ed)*. 1986;292(6516):318–320. doi:10.1136/bmj.292.6516.318

Krahn, G. L., Robinson, A., Murray, A., and Havercamp, S. It's time to reconsider how we define health: Perspective from disability and chronic condition. *Disabil Health J*. 2021;14(4). doi:10.1016/j.dhjo.2021.101129

Pamuk, E., Makuc, D., Heck, K., Reuben, C., and Lochner, K. *Socioeconomic Status and Health Chartbook*. US National Center for Health Statistics; 1998.

Saracci, R. The World Health Organization needs to reconsider its definition of health. *BMJ*. 1997;314(7091):1409–1410. doi:10.1136/bmj.314.7091.1409

Van Druten, V. P., Bartels, E. A., van de Mheen, D., de Vries, E., Kerckhoffs, A. P. M., and Nahar-Van Venrooij, L. M. W. Concepts of health in different contexts: A scoping review. *BMC Health Serv Res*. 2022;22:389. doi:10.1186/s12913-022-07702-2

CHAPTER 2

Understanding Health as a Wicked Problem

2.0 Introduction

The problems we face in dealing with health and especially the delivery of healthcare and health services are diverse. Moreover, these problems are charged with multiple stakeholder interests derived from information that is complex, complicated, and even confusing. Horst Rittel, a professor at the University of California at Berkley, first described these problems as belonging to a distinct type of problem that cannot be solved but can only be tamed (Churchman, 1967). Rittel used the term "wicked" to describe such problems.

2.1 Health Is a Wicked Problem

Wicked problems are multifarious. They are often symptoms of larger problems, without definitive resolutions or stopping rules,[1] and may lead to cascading outcomes without a clear trace back to the original problem (Rittel and Webber, 1973).

In health, wicked problems are more the norm than the exception. Problems in health are both complicated and complex. They are often insolvable, and they lead us to recognize that what we perceive to be the issue is often a symptom of a deeper predicament. The fundamental factors of health – physical, mental, emotional, spiritual, and social – contribute to the wickedness of problems in health because they add to the complexity of the problem.

The complex problem is a function of the interaction between multiple factors (Poli, 2013), wherein each factor contributes non-linearly to the outcome and, in most circumstances, demonstrates a disproportionate contribution to the outcome(s). Complex problems lead to the establishment of outcomes that are viewed more as a system of events than as a unique entity. Complex problems have depth and dimensionality that is neither obvious nor capable of exploration. Given the ubiquitous tangential characteristics that impact complex problems, it *should* be expected that multiple solutions will be raised to resolve the problem without considering the magnitude of the complexity.

DOI: 10.4324/9781003474777-2

2.2 Contrasting Complicated With Complexity

In the *complicated* problem, we find that the pieces which comprise the whole are recognizable and have a proportionate contribution to the outcome. In a *complicated* problem, the messiness can be ordered and can thereby contribute to a permanent resolution to the problem.

> **Complicated problems are not wicked problems.**

That doesn't mean complicated problems are easy to solve, but it does mean that complicated problems lack complexity.

Endeavoring to eradicate all potential calamities associated with epidemics or pandemics is a wicked problem. In wicked problems, we accept that there are no stopping rules (Rittel and Webber, 1973). This means that we cannot know when our efforts to eradicate the causes of epidemics have been successful. This is primarily because we lack the complete knowledge of factors that lead to the introduction of new diseases into society. Likewise, we must respect the complexity of human activity and the interaction between humans and the precursors to disease emergence.

Often, the complicatedness and the complexity of a problem are so intertwined that it may be impossible to separate the resolvable complicated bits from the non-resolvable complex elements. For example, establishing rules to control the spread of the COVID-19 pandemic is not a wicked problem. Previous evidence from studies on approaches to reduce disease spread provides ample support for methods to control viral load and spread (Ellwanger et al., 2021). Establishing the rules deemed necessary to control disease spread is a complicated problem. It is messy, and it necessitates a rules-based approach that will cause consternation within the population, but the rules can be organized and recommended. The challenge to this approach is that it may not be possible to enforce controls on societal movement that are intended to ensure a reduction in the risk of disease.

Controlling the likelihood of an epidemic and, worse yet, a pandemic, is a wicked problem because of the complexity of the issues that arise within a population and which can lead to negative outcomes (Kerr and Glantz, 2020). Managing the population to conform to the suggested rules intended to prevent the spread of the virus is a wicked problem because it requires that the population accept the responsibilities required to make substantial changes to their daily routines. The introduction of rules and regulations implicitly assumes both acceptance and compliance. Complexity is compounded in some societies when the rules are viewed as restrictions and are therefore perceived to contravene freedoms. Assuming that the entire population would conform to the suggested measures to control viral spread and subsequently viral load of COVID-19 was shown to be unlikely. For many governments, their best efforts to control the spread of the COVID-19 pandemic required the imposition of rules to maintain a positive state of physical health for the general public. As such, governments around the world followed the advice of the World Health Organization and especially the obligations to which most countries agreed to uphold as signatories of "The Right to the Highest Attainable Standard of Health" (Montel et al., 2020). For the most part, this meant that governments published and distributed specific guidelines such as the requirements to wear masks, maintain a distance between people of some 2 meters, and avoid congregating in large groups – indoors, especially for prolonged periods of time. The belief and obvious outcome was that when we demonstrated contrary behaviors, such as congregating in large groups without wearing a mask and ignoring the considerations for social distancing, we increased the risk of viral spread, and concomitantly, the *incidence rate*[2] of the disease also increased, as expected. However, when we complied with the suggested restrictions and adhered to the guidelines, we demonstrated a greater likelihood to be successful in controlling the spread of the case rate or, as the vernacular suggested, *flattened the curve* – and thereby moved society toward resolving the disease spread problem.

> **Complicated problems can be solved; wicked problems are not solved but resolved.**

As noted by Rittel and Webber (1973), with wicked problems, any perception of a solution to a defined element of the problem is a one-time shot – with no opportunity to learn from the outcome because each new wicked problem will be different. Creating a schedule to distribute the COVID-19 vaccine and similar public health vaccination programs designed to reduce the risk of disease *prevalence*[3] are, again, not wicked problems but can be considered complicated problems. By creating a regulatory strategy that is consistent with government procedures and capabilities, we can accomplish widespread distribution of vaccinations and increase disease prevention.

Combining immunization programs with public health promotion strategies, in general, can enhance the positive physical, mental, and social health of populations and, in so doing, have an indirect effect on financial health personally and an overall positive effect on the economy. For example, promoting and adopting behaviors that include practicing positive hygiene that blocks pathogens from entering the body will reduce the risk of illness development. Far too often, health promoters have espoused the messages to practice essential health behaviors but repeatedly to an indifferent public. No doubt that you have heard or seen public health messaging that reminds us to wash our hands regularly with soap and water – especially after using the toilet – to avoid touching our face, to cover our mouth when sneezing or coughing, along with direct messages to practice safe sex – specifically to use a condom. Moreover, since the pandemic, we can add the increased frequency with which we are told to avoid social gatherings (including work and play) if you are dealing with ill-health such as seasonal flu or infectious diseases, because adopting such behaviors can reduce the risk of disease spread. Yet, as often, the message has been disregarded and dismissed without recourse.

Human behaviors are complex and multifactored. Culture, geography, perceived need, desires, and personal preferences are among the many factors that each contribute independently and interactively to drive behaviors. Such factors cannot be controlled. However, as a society, we strive to reduce the negative consequences of resultant behaviors through regulations and laws. In the COVID-19 pandemic, we observed that despite the best efforts of public health officials to control the spread of the pandemic by instituting rules and regulations, societies and government leaders around the world resisted and demonstrated their disapproval of such constraints on personal freedoms. In some countries, the consequences of disobeying such laws were extremely severe, while in other countries, the lack of enforcement and contrary views between government leaders and public health experts led to super-spreader events and, subsequently, an increase in *case fatality rates*[4] within the specific geographic area and time period. At our best, we can only reduce the risk of epidemics and pandemics by reducing the risk factors – those behaviors or conditions that lead to the emergence or spread of disease or infirmity.

This satisfies another criterion for wicked problems – that is, we cannot achieve a true-versus-false outcome, but the outcome of a wicked problem is deemed to be a good versus a bad outcome. If we practice all behaviors that reduce incidence risk, then we have done well, and we will have attained a good outcome. However, if our behaviors lead to conditions that increase the incidence risk, then we have done poorly, and the result is a bad outcome.

In health, as in other disciplines, the accepted rhetoric is that wicked problems are rarely solved despite the numerous approaches that introduce systematic and innovative strategies for success. For example, some researchers suggest that wicked problems can be resolved with a groupthink or networked approach that builds on collective intelligence (Williams, 2023) in which knowledge evolves and is shared from individuals to teams (Elia and Margherita, 2018).

Despite that Rittel and Webber suggested that no criteria exist to evaluate strategies for the resolution of wicked problems, Head and Alford (2015) proposed that by considering the type of wicked problem being investigated, there may be a spectrum of approaches that can be consistently used to address wicked problems. To this end, Head and Alford (2015) described three types of problems which can be recognized in various processing capacities. The first is considered to be the tame problem – here, both the problem and the suggested solution to the problem are manageable by the decision-maker. Next is a basic wicked problem. In this situation, the problem appears to be clear or at least well understood, but the solution to the problem is unclear. Head and Alford attribute this lack of clarity to the inability to discern a cause–effect relationship that underlies the problem. The third type of problem they proposed is one in which neither the problem definition nor the relevant solution to the ill-defined problem is clear. This latter type of problem is often described as one you just can't put your finger on or just can't wrap your brain around.

However, Head and Alford did not buy into the non-resolution mantra of wicked problems and rather suggested that taking a broader-thinking approach to unpacking the wicked problem may lead to success in processing a problem resolution. The approaches suggested by these researchers include not only taking a more holistic approach but also incorporating practices that are not traditional to the environment in which the problem-solving exercise is performed. That is, Head and Alford suggested that using collaborative and coordinated approaches can lead to complementary thinking that takes advantage of input from across a cooperative group that has emerged to respond to the problem-solving task. In this way, the traditional hierarchy of decision-making is dismantled, and in its place emerges a shared contribution of strategies to address the issues that underlie the problem.

In addition to addressing wicked problems using different strategies, others have promoted specific tools to tame the wicked problem. For example, Horn and Weber (2007) discussed *resolution mapping*, in which groups of individuals work collectively and begin by first evaluating the problem and then combining their strategies based on the evaluation of outcomes to form stepwise tactics. In so doing, this approach *creates a map*, or a distinct pathway that can be followed to resolve perceived a problem and produce a desirable outcome.

Still others suggest that to solve a wicked problem, we need to combine expertise from diverse and disparate partners, as in creating a culture between experts and deep thinkers from across the fabric of a society. Consider, for example, a group of individuals drawn from higher education establishments collaborating with community-based individuals that can draw on life experiences in an applied interdisciplinary approach which takes advantage of the shared intelligence of multiple stakeholders and brings together seasoned senior professionals with energetic and enthusiastic novices (Cantor et al., 2015). In effect, this would evolve to a network of contributors and represent a diverse cohort within a community.

While the many suggestions for successful resolution of wicked problems provide distinctive strategies, the dependency on a network approach appears to be the most consistent recommendation. As noted by Weber and Khademian (2008), the network has the potential to facilitate communication in which knowledge can be shared, and outcomes can be based on an emergence of collaborative capacity.

Given the criteria that define wicked problems as being unique and relentless, no single problem-solving strategy will be considered sufficiently complete. Moreover, the accepted mantra by many who recognize the futility in attempting to solve a wicked problem is that rather than solving a wicked problem, at best, we can only tame the wicked problem (Camillus, 2008), which is to resolve[5] the wicked problem.

The reason we can only tame a wicked problem is because we seldom agree on the starting point – a term Xiang (2013) referred to as "indeterminacy in problem formulation." That is, because of the diversity of backgrounds and specific interests of those trying to solve the wicked problem, we fail to develop a concise and comprehensive statement of the problem and thereby cannot establish clear and definitive criteria to solve the problem. This conundrum leads to a second, insurmountable barrier to successfully solving wicked problems. That is, since we cannot put our finger on the problem, we cannot establish valid and reliable measurement outcomes. Xiang (2013) calls this characteristic "non-definitiveness in problem solution."

Wicked problems deal with multiple perspectives – and as noted by Rittel and Webber (1973), a critical feature of a wicked problem is that striving to solve the wicked problem may lead to identifying new issues that expose emergent problems, each as unsolvable and often with solutions that are worse than the initial wicked problem. Yet conceding to the challenges of wicked problems is not an option. On the contrary, just as there are multiple dimensions to wicked problems, there are multiple approaches to taming wicked problems, or at least to recognizing the wickedness of the problem and creating strategies to work around the problem.

In health, as we consider the methods by which we can resolve wicked problems, we often consider the cadre of next generation researchers and policymakers who will be tasked with the responsibility to tackle evolving as well as stagnant wicked problems. In this regard, there are emerging conversations to rethink the training of graduate students and young scientists to deal with the ever-expanding recognition of wicked problems. For example, Kawa et al. (2021) offer a salient argument on the need for disciplines to provide explicit recognition of wicked problems throughout the education training process, which would provide structure and organization to the methods by which wicked problems can be handled. The authors argue for a mind-shift in the training of graduate programs that would push students and young faculty out of their cognate disciplines and into pursuing transdisciplinary projects that expand new ways of thinking.

Problems that arise within the realm of planetary health are examples of the need for transdisciplinary schemes that demonstrate the value of versatility required to chip away at the larger wicked problem. Planetary health studies the relationship between changes to the entire planet that result in specific effects to the natural systems of Earth's evolution and the influence of these effects on human health and well-being globally. Planetary health is not restricted to the physical Earth but to the combined elements within the biosphere along with the physical systems that influence the biosphere (Pongsiri et al., 2019).

When senior researchers and academic leaders actively engage, build, and support creative learning environments that foster new communities of practice, wicked problems are more likely to become common pursuits. The actions associated with extreme climate events and the effects on planetary health exemplify the need to change the way we respond to these wicked problems and demonstrate the value of approaching the problems from a transdisciplinary perspective. Moreover, when senior researchers, academics, and thought leaders explicitly discount the stigma of productivity and competition in research, especially as criteria for employment, then tackling wicked problems will become commonplace among researchers who participate in transdisciplinary research teams and can thereby address more aspects within the Gestalt of the problem.

Addressing the methods by which wicked problems can be solved or resolved has led to the development of emerging schools of thought, two of which are implementation science and complexity science. As Lavery (2018) noted, implementation science emerged as a method by which we might address the challenges that establish the wickedness of problems. And Braithwaite and colleagues (2018) described complexity science as a method (not a theory) by which the dynamic properties of problems are viewed within a systems approach. It's not a linear system or a system that removes or discounts the complexity of the properties that characterize the problem, because, as Braithwaite mentioned, others have reminded us that eliminating or reducing complexity is the default approach that humans use to understand complexity. Rather, as Kawa and coworkers (2021) suggest, consider the elements of the problem to include the socio-political nature of the wicked problem and, in so doing, expand the transdisciplinary nature of the roots of the wickedness.

Both implementation science and complexity science are fundamental to providing approaches for dealing with wicked problems, be those problems in health or in other areas. Likewise, both are emerging disciplines with different underlying philosophical approaches. For example, implementation science, which is described as an approach to closing the gap between evidence and action, is an area that provides the potential structure required to resolve wicked problems (Young-Wolff et al., 2016; Lobb and Colditz, 2013). In comparison, complexity science was described by Phelan (2001) as a way of knowing based on the methods of science. Complexity science, according to Churruca et al. (2019), describes systems that may be messy and at the "edge of chaos." Complexity science advances issues using approaches that are transferable across disciplines, and hence, complexity science schemas are used in the social sciences to understand financial and economic systems and in the health sciences to understand health services delivery systems along with the more traditional applications to the physical sciences as in understanding chaos.

2.3 Contrasting Implementation Science and Complexity Science

According to Lobb and Colditz (2013), implementation science evolved in the United States during the decade of the 60s because of planning, execution, and evaluation of national initiatives designed to support population health. In implementation science, the efforts of researchers, planners, practitioners, and policymakers from diverse and disparate disciplines are combined to consolidate ideas and perspectives in a struggle to move evidence-based interventions into practice. Eventually, these practices spawn policies that help to ensure the sustainability of best practices for positive population health outcomes.

Implementation science is a discipline which can build on the collaborative capacity of a network to resolve wicked problems. Activities that begin, typically as ideas for case studies or as use-case scenarios, expand to become interventions that are implemented in real-world applications. In implementation science, the applications are based on appropriate evidence. Here, the term *appropriate* is critical to the conversation because the evidence must be reliable: consistent, valid, and generalizable to ensure that the real-world practice can be optimized. According to Lobb and Colditz (2013), the importance of ensuring that the evidence upon which interventions are based is both reliable – that is, to demonstrate stability through a process of test and retest – and valid, applying what made sense in theory to enhance the strength of the emerging evidence.

Implementation science is optimized when collaborators, as in a network of diverse-minded individuals, can maximize their contribution to resolving issues. Implementation science will provide solutions and strategies for complicated and messy problems, but the approaches of implementation science are most effective when the focus is on wicked problems. To this end, researchers, planners, practitioners, and policymakers need to understand the limitations of the resolution and identify the best methods by which the network can tame wicked problems.

As noted by Churruca and colleagues (2019), complexity science is an approach by which we can make sense of the multifactorial non-linearity that underlies wicked problems. Complexity science is pervasive in health, but because it is implicit throughout many applications, it may not be regarded as a modus operandi to respond to wicked problems. Issues that arise as health-related problems are often dealt with immediately. This does not mean that the problem is resolved nor that the correct approach has been taken. Rather, this implies that as a collective, we often jump into action to produce an evidence-based notion, constructed on a linear approach, to make sense of the problem and with the intention to solve the problem as we perceive it to be (Petrie and Peters, 2020).

Complexity science has a rich toolbox (Mohammadi, 2020) that may be underused as an explicit methodology by which to address wicked problems in health and, more importantly, in the fundamental disciplines upon which the delivery of elements to enhance the health of a population is comprised – i.e., health education, health promotion, health policy, and health services. One consideration that may help us to explain why we disregard a foray into complexity science approaches is the uncertainty that must be accepted in approaching wicked problems from a complexity perspective. According to Petrie and Peters (2020) and Rogers et al. (2013), to become more comfortable in using complexity science to address wicked problems, we should consider three fundamental approaches that are important to the way we think about and deal with issues of complexity (aka the wickedness of emerging problems). The first approach is openness – which is related to open-mindedness about ideas/opinions and developing an acceptance of emergent notions. The second approach is to establish situational awareness – which is described as the ability to recognize diversity and relationships that could exist. The third approach is to recognize the need to respect the restraint/action paradox – which is described as losing the fear of failure and accepting the pervasiveness of risk to embrace complexity.

Even though health interventions are evidence based, many will underperform, be harmful to recipients, be dismissed by professionals, or be de-implemented for use in real-world health applications. Such events are not necessarily because the interventions were developed on a lack of evidence, but as likely, because emerging conditions within cohorts of recipients and changes in the dynamics of populations differ from those which existed when the original information was established. Evidence-based interventions can be passed over for use because of the complexity of the system into which they would be used. Similarly, because the intended application of the selected implementation is designed to resolve a wicked problem within the larger body of health, the critical mass of informed individuals needed to carry out the appropriate implementation is lacking.

Norton and Chambers (2020) stated that interventions are de-implemented because they fail to meet the necessary rigor of evaluative methods to ensure patient safety, maintain public trust, and reduce economic burden. Overcoming the wickedness of problems in health requires that evidence-based interventions are valid, requiring precision and accuracy of purpose. Evidence-based programs that are designed to resolve wicked problems in health must be relevant, or they will lack the capacity to be generalizable. Failing to generalize will reduce the potential for spread and scale of the resolution beyond the original cohort(s) upon which the original work was established. Preferably, there needs to be an explicit transfer of knowledge to larger target populations. When wicked problems are decidedly resolved, this is generally by a one-time approach. Therefore, the ability to demonstrate repeatability within the same cohort over time is not possible. Rather, measures of consistency are limited to reflecting initial group dynamics and not reproducible beyond the local original cases.

Whereas complexity science provides an approach to understanding and identifying if not defining the wicked problem, implementation science has emerged as being synonymous with knowledge translation (Young, 2015). Interventions derived from evidence-based applications in real-world settings are introduced to problems in health with an intention to provide resolutions and improvements, regardless of whether the problems are complex or complicated. Poverty is a health problem; poverty is a social determinant of health; poverty is a wicked problem (Spicker, 2016) because it is multidimensional, without a clear description of the issues that need to be resolved. Poverty is nuanced, it does not follow a mechanistic system of stopping rules and trace-back pathways. The study of poverty has provided tremendous volumes of information upon which knowledge is constructed, but despite our best efforts, poverty is an insurmountable health problem that will not be eradicated.

If you live below the expected minimum annual income threshold, also known as a low-income cut-off (LICO), within a given country, then you are most likely a member of the lowest of the socioeconomic classes within that country and may even be considered to exist in poverty. This bottom of the socioeconomic classes is the class that is becoming increasingly identified as the definite cause of lower life expectancy, increased likelihood to experience violence, and having a corresponding relationship with adverse childhood events leading to chronic disease outcomes later in life (Gupta et al., 2007). The complexity of poverty as a problem that warrants strategies that not only deal with resolving the financial constraints that families in poverty experience, but the resolution must also recognize the social dimension of poverty which includes cultural shame and stigma.

In 2018, the federal government of Canada proposed the Canadian Poverty Reduction strategy Duclos (2018) as a set of priorities to lift citizens out of poverty. This was an implementation strategy designed specifically to build on the knowledge that reducing poverty requires more than merely providing a stable income. While the strategy recognized the multidimensional dynamics of poverty, such as the importance of establishing food security, as well as providing affordable and safe housing, employment security, and education to improve literacy, along with provisions for child support, establishing financial security through a basic income guarantee is one of the most important contributions a government can make to enable its citizenry to overcome the barriers to health.

Such enabling strategies are designed to address poverty both at a national level and by working directly with local communities in states, provinces, territories, and the governments of the Indigenous Peoples: First Nations, Metis, and Inuit. These strategies build momentum by providing access to better housing, food security, education, and childcare, to name but a few of the benefits. If these strategies can be maintained in a non-partisan consortium of stakeholders and decision-makers, and if the decisions of the National Advisory Council on Poverty are respected and incorporated into policy, the implementation of such strategies could impact the wickedness of poverty and help to resolve this wicked health problem.

In health, and especially with regard to population health issues, Jayasinghe (2011) described our typical approach to problem-solving as being mechanistic and often following the criteria of reductionism (that is, reducing a problem to basic elements), linearity (assuming that there is a straightforward approach to problem-solving), and hierarchical power distribution, whereby the approach to the issues of the problem have a step-down or central core heuristic that ensures transfer of information from a central power repository to a solution. Rogers et al. (2013) concluded that complexity science applications require a new tactic in addressing issues. Adopting a complexity science method demands that we break out of our traditional linear thinking or mechanistic approach – that we extend our considerations to problem resolution methods beyond the linearity of reductionist strategies. To address the complexity of wicked problems, such as those which are central to health, and the effects of various systems on health of populations, we need to reconsider the patterns of our problem-solving behaviors to acknowledge the diversity of possible solutions and the dynamics of problems which we address as active participants.

2.4 Conclusion

If we reconsider our approach to health issues from a complexity science approach, we will be more likely to approach our wicked problems not by looking for a breakdown in a linear flow or identifying a malfunction of one or more parts of the machinery within a system that influences the gestalt of our health. Rather, if we reconsider our approach to complex problem resolution by placing less emphasis on mechanistic thinking, then we will reduce our expectations that the issue can be resolved by modifying the central power resource within the hierarchy. If we adopt a complexity science approach, we will accept that the issues do not lie with a central administrator within a system but that there will be integration of systems that contribute at a fundamental level. Likewise, we will accept that there are nuances within the systems that cannot be reduced to simple parts. To accept the wickedness of problems is to accept the complexity of problems, and therefore, we must reconsider the approach to problem resolution.

As Jayasinghe suggests, our approach to resolving wicked problems can consider that health and thereby health outcomes are part of an open system that functions because of a web of causation and not merely an oversimplified stimulus–response system. Issues that arise within a cohort, a population, or a specific context are multifactorial and emerge as a function of the interaction and integration of a variety of inputs, some of which are measurable and some of which cannot be measured or explained, even if they are suspected to exist.

Just as there are no stopping rules in dealing with wicked problems, there are no fixed limits or pre-designated patterns that form the basis for the appropriate heuristic methods applied in wicked problem resolution. Health is a wicked problem that necessitates the evolution of our thinking, our behavior, and thus our approach to problem resolution.

2.4.1 Discussion Questions

1 The core element of a wicked problem is that it is more than complicated in that it is complex. How does complex differ from complicated? What other adjectives can be used to describe wicked problems? How does health fit the definition of a wicked problem?
2 We stated that wicked problems are ubiquitous in health. If we wish to transform health systems, in light of the wickedness that besets health services delivery, how might we approach resolving wicked problems in health?

Notes

1 A stopping rule is a distinct statement used in areas of decision-making when a procedure, process, game, or system is to end. For example, in clinical trials, a stopping rule might be to end the trial when an outcome has been achieved and there is no need to collect additional data.
2 The number of new cases observed within a given time period. Incidence rate has time as a specific factor which indicates that it is a rate and not merely a proportion.
3 Prevalence is not a rate but a ratio – a proportion. The term *prevalence* refers to the ratio of cases of a disease or outcome relative to all of those individuals that are at risk for the disease or outcome.
4 Case fatality rate refers to the number of people who die during a time period in relation to all of those who were diagnosed with the condition of interest (disease) during the time period.

5 In the context of a wicked problem, the term *resolve* implies that we have settled on an approach to handle the problem that is neither fixed nor rigid but is open to continued scrutiny and adjustment as evidence emerges.

References

Braithwaite, J., Churruca, K., Long, J. C., Ellis, L. A., & Herkes, J. (2018). When complexity science meets implementation science: A theoretical and empirical analysis of systems change. *BMC Medicine*, 16, 63. https://doi.org/10.1186/s12916-018-1057-z

Camillus, J. C. (2008). Strategy as a wicked problem. *Harvard Business Review*, 1–9.

Cantor, A., DeLauer, V., Martin, D., & Rogan, J. (2015). Training interdisciplinary "wicked problem" solvers: Applying lessons from HERO in community-based research experiences for undergraduates. *Journal of Geography in Higher Education*, 39(3), 407–419. https://doi.org/10.1080/03098265.2015.1048508

Churchman, C. W. (1967). Guest editorial: Wicked problems. *Management Science*, 14(4), B141–B142.

Churruca, K., Pomare, C., Ellis, L. A., Long, J. C., & Braithwaite, J. (2019). The influence of complexity: A bibliometric analysis of complexity science in healthcare. *BMJ Open*, 9, e027308. https://doi.org/10.1136/bmjopen-2018-027308

Duclos, J.-Y. (2018). *Canadian poverty reduction strategy – What we heard about poverty so far.* (Cat. No.: Em12-48/2018E-PDF). ISSN: 978-0-660-26905-4. Retrieved from canada.ca/publicentre-ESDC on 9 May 2024.

Elia, G., & Margherita, A. (2018). Can we solve wicked problems? A conceptual framework and a collective intelligence system to support problem analysis and solution design for complex social issues. *Technological Forecasting and Social Change*, 133, 279–286.

Ellwanger, J. H., Veiga, A. B. G., Kaminski, V. L., Valverde-Villegas, J. M., Freitas, A. W. Q., & Chies, J. A. B. (2021). Control and prevention of infectious diseases from a one health perspective. *Genetics and Molecular Biology*, 44(1 Suppl. 1), e20200256. https://doi.org/10.1590/1678-4685-GMB-2020-0256

Gupta, R., de Wit, M., & McKeown, D. (2007). The impact of poverty on the current and future health status of children. *Paediatrics & Child Health*, 12(8), 667–672.

Head, B. W., & Alford, J. (2015). Wicked problems: Implications for public policy and management. *Administration & Society*, 47(6), 711–739. https://doi.org/10.1177/0095399713481601

Horn, R., & Weber, R. P. (2007). *New tools for resolving wicked problems: Mess mapping and resolution mapping processes* (Volume 1.2, 31 pp.). MacroVU(r), Inc. and Strategy Kinetics, LLC.

Jayasinghe, S. (2011). Conceptualizing population health: From mechanistic thinking to complexity science. *Emerging Themes in Epidemiology*, 8, 2. https://doi.org/10.1186/1742-7622-8-2

Kawa, N. C., Arceño, M. A., Goeckner, R., Hunter, C. E., Rhue, S. J., Scaggs, S. A., Biwer, M. E., Downey, S. S., Field, J. S., Gremillion, K., McCorriston, J., Willow, A., Newton, E., & Moritz, M. (2021). Training wicked scientists for a world of wicked problems. *Humanities and Social Sciences Communications*, 8, 189. https://doi.org/10.1057/s41599-021-00871-1

Kerr, D., & Glantz, N. (2020). Diabetes, like COVID-19, is a wicked problem. *The Lancet*, 8. www.thelancet.com/diabetes-endocrinology; https://doi.org/10.1016/S2213-8587(20)30312-0

Lavery, J. V. (2018). Wicked problems, community engagement, and the need for an implementation science for research ethics. *Journal of Medical Ethics*, 44, 163–164.

Lobb, R., & Colditz, G. (2013). Implementation science and its application to population health. *Annual Review of Public Health*, 34, 235–251.

Mohammadi, N. K. (2020). Diffusion of complexity science into health promotion research and practice: Foundations for a complex future. *Health Promotion International*, 1–7.

Montel, L., Kapilashrami, A., Coleman, M. P., & Allemani, C. (2020). The right to health in times of pandemic: What can we learn from the UK's response to the COVID-19 outbreak? *Health and Human Rights*, 22(2), 227–241.

Norton, W. E., & Chambers, D. A. (2020). Unpacking the complexities of de-implementing inappropriate health interventions. *Implementation Science*, 15(1), 2. https://doi.org/10.1186/s13012-019-0960-9

Petrie, S., & Peters, P. (2020). Untangling complexity as a health determinant: Wicked problems in healthcare. *Health Science Inquiry*, 11, 131–135.

Phelan, S. (2001). What is complexity science, really? *Emergence*, 3(1), 120–136.

Poli, J. (2013). A note on the difference between complicated and complex social systems. *CADMUS: Promoting Leadership in Thought That Leads to Action*, 2(1), 142–147.

Pongrisi, M. J., Bickersteth, S., Colon, C., DeFries, R., Dhaliwal, M., Georgeson, L., Haines, A., Linou, N., Murray, V., Naeem, S., Small, R., & Ungvari, J. (2019). Planetary health: From concept to decisive action. *The Lancet*, 3(10), E402–E404.

Rittel, H., & Webber, M. (1973). Dilemmas in a general theory of planning. *Policy Sciences*, 4, 155–169. https://doi.org/10.1007/BF01405730

Rogers, K. H., Luton, R., Biggs, H., Biggs, R. (Oonsie), Blignaut, S., Choles, A. G., Palmer, C. G., & Tangwe, P. (2013). Fostering complexity thinking in action research for change in social – ecological systems. *Ecology and Society*, 18(2). www.jstor.org/stable/26269310

Spicker, P. (2016). *Poverty as a wicked problem* (CROP poverty brief, no. 35). Bergen: CROP Secretariat. www.crop.org/viewfile.aspx?id=1062

Weber, E. P., & Khademian, A. M. (2008). Wicked problems, knowledge challenges, and collaborative capacity builders in network settings. *Public Administration Review*, 334–349.

Williams, A. E. (2023). Are wicked problems a lack of general collective intelligence? *AI & Society*, 38, 343–348. https://doi.org/10.1007/s00146-021-01297-8

Xiang, W.-N. (2013). Editorial (working with wicked problems in socio-ecological systems: Awareness, acceptance, and adaptation). *Landscape and Urban Planning*, 110, 1–4.

Young, A. M. (2015). Solving the wicked problem of hospital malnutrition. *Nutrition & Dietetics*, 72(3), 200–204.

Young-Wolff, K. C., Kotz, K., & McCaw, B. (2016). Transforming the health care response to intimate partner violence: Addressing "wicked problems". *JAMA: The Journal of the American Medical Association*, 315(23), 2517–2518. https://doi.org/10.1001/jama.2016.4837

Epidemiological Applications for Human Health

3.0 Introduction

In primary healthcare research, benchtop studies are supported by randomized clinical trials, and surveillance systems are designed to monitor events that impact populations, while program planners design evaluation strategies of interventions. Prospective and retrospective cohort comparisons are used to evaluate research hypotheses, secondary data analyses recycle information to enhance knowledge, and meta-analytic approaches and systematic reviews help to establish or challenge the validity of assumptions.

Many elements in the delivery of healthcare draw upon the accumulated evidence that has been provided through the application of these primary, secondary, and tertiary research methods; and together, these various methods have created an abundance of essential evidence to support programs to enhance health services, healthcare delivery, and health interventions at the population, community, and individual levels. Such evidence is essential to decision-making about condition-specific treatments and strategies that ensure prevention or protection from adverse health stimuli and extend beyond merely physical health.

A fundamental tool in the process of evidence gathering for health research and decision-making related to health policy formation and program planning, especially in public health applications, is epidemiology. Simply defined as *the study of* (*ology*) health conditions *on* or *upon* (*epi*) *people* (*demos*), epidemiology is multifunctional as a robust methodology for providing the essential evidence in decision-making related to the general health and well-being of our planet and all its constituents.

Applications of epidemiological methods are used extensively in understanding human health and the implications of our lived experiences to achieve specific health outcomes. A mainstay of epidemiological methods is the collection of secure data, which is essential to the process of information gathering for the purposes of developing knowledge. Data is the grist for the mill to provide the evidence for health policy formation and decision-making in the development, planning, promotion, and delivery of health services.

DOI: 10.4324/9781003474777-3

The application of epidemiological methods based on sound research design and statistical principles in the investigation of health conditions has provided extensive support to decision-making among those who form the cadre of multidisciplinary healthcare practitioners. By providing timely access to high-quality relevant information about trends and behaviors at a population level, and by establishing systems of health surveillance and tools to measure health service compliance, and data from diagnostic outcomes, practitioners, researchers, and policymakers can make informed decisions that impact the health of populations, communities, and ultimately individuals.

Epidemiological methods include the development and use of health surveillance systems, conducting field investigations, designing and implementing analytic studies, evaluating programs, and establishing data linkages across databases and registries. Although these applications will differ across health professionals, the ability to understand and use such methods at a basic skill level is essential. Specifically, individuals working in primary and allied fields of human health will be expected to continuously maintain and upgrade their ability to read and interpret health reports at a local, regional, national, and international level. To this end, health professionals will be expected to ensure data quality, especially when reporting on trends and tendencies of health outcomes using descriptive methodologies. Many will need to upgrade their skills so that they can conduct basic statistical analyses that determine the importance of observed outcomes and both help plan and manage basic databases of information.

There is little doubt that the COVID-19 pandemic has shown the relevance of epidemiological methods. Moreover, because of daily reporting of rates of morbidity (illness) and mortality (death), there was a growing interest amongst the public to understand epidemiological methods and the application of these methods to determine the dynamics of the coronavirus disease.[1] In the future, the public will continue to expect that health professionals demonstrate appropriate communication skills in knowledge translation and knowledge dissemination so that they can rely on the important and accurate messaging that is delivered en masse.

Health professionals will be the gatekeepers between the public and the scientists to ensure that evidence which has been synthesized from various procedures is explained in clear and concise terms. Health professionals will be required to apply that which has been learned from analyses of surveillance system outcomes to program planning, policy formation, and decision-making that will help to protect the public and prevent adverse health consequences while optimizing resource allocation.

In this regard, the use of epidemiological methods is imperative to enable the integration of evidence into real-world decision-making and to the evaluation of the efficacy of applied practices to maintain and enhance human health. Among the fundamental tenets of epidemiological methods are time, place, and person (Fox et al., 2022). In developing our understanding of the occurrence of conditions of interest relative to human health outcomes, each of these tenets provides valuable evidence in our decision-making processes. For example, time is a fundamental variable (Osterholm and Hedberg, 2015) because it can be used as the denominator to calculate incidence rates, which provides the number of new cases observed within a defined time period. Equally, time is essential to the estimate of prevalence, which indicates the total number of cases at a specific time point. Additionally, time provides the estimate of duration for the presence of conditions of interest.

Similarly, place and person are equally important in providing evidence in the application of epidemiological methods. Place can refer to global geography or local communities and, in so doing, can help to visualize both the location of conditions of interest as well as to illustrate the spread and scale of conditions of interest. Likewise, *person* is a term that helps to define the cohort that is affected by the condition of interest, and when studied in detail along with place, it helps to uncover other restrictions within society that influence outcomes. For example, while the three tenets of time, place, and person are the first step in understanding outbreaks, a deeper dive into *persons in place* can show the effects of various conditions of interest on the human health gestalt for marginalized cohorts and communities in a region. As noted by (Wachtler et al., 2020), individuals that are deemed to have a low socioeconomic status are more likely to die or succumb to the condition of interest. This contention was brought to light early in the epidemiological measurement of the COVID-19 pandemic, when Wachtler and colleagues reported that marginalized individuals were more likely to be infected by the SARS-CoV-2 virus. Later findings by Udell et al. (2022) supported Wachtler and colleagues by showing that there was a greater likelihood of contracting the virus when demonstrating specific risk factors such as being male, living in low-income neighborhoods, being part of an ethnic or racial community, being an immigrant, or having hypertension or diabetes. Specifically, Udell and coworkers (2022) reported that individuals with at least two risk factors for SARS-CoV-2 were slightly less than twice as likely to become infected, while having three risk factors increased the likelihood to three times as likely to be infected, and having four or more risk factors increased the likelihood to be infected to nearly five times compared to individuals at lower risk levels.

3.1 On the Importance of the Experiment

One of the fundamental principles of scientific inquiry is the experiment.

In its simplest form, an experiment is a research process using a planned comparison in which an outcome can be attributed to a condition or conditions of interest.

At the outset of the experiment's design, we establish a hypothesis. The hypothesis is the statement of expectation related to the experiment's outcome, and thus we say that it is a method by which we can test our hypothesis or our statement of expectation.

The elements that make up an experiment are referred to as variables, and variables are simply defined as containers that hold information. As we dive deeper into the meaning and applications of experimental research, we can categorize the variables into different forms. In a simple experiment, we may have two types of variables – the input variables and the outcome variables. For example, consider the simple equation $Y = X$. Here, Y is the label of the variable that represents an outcome, while X is the label of the variable representing the input. In research applications, we say that the output variable Y is dependent on the input variable X.

In epidemiological applications, the information that is contained in the variables Y and X is data, where data can take many forms. Often, we think about data in a digital sense, and of course, this is appropriate when we are attempting to work through mathematical calculations. However, data is much more than a set of numerical observations. Data can be images, sounds, frequencies, oral histories, videos, or any information that contextualizes collected facts. Data is essential to describing the circumstances of interest and telling the stories of outcomes and events.

In the experiment, we set specific conditions for the data contained in the variables that comprise it. Again, considering a simple experiment, we call the outcome variable the dependent variable because it is dependent on the characteristics of the input variable. Similarly, we refer to the input variable as the independent variable because it is not dependent on other influencing factors but rather is controlled by the experimenter.

In a simple cause-and-effect experiment, we identify the cause as the independent variable and the effect as the outcome or dependent variable. Using mathematical notation to represent the cause-and-effect relationship as shown here, Y is the outcome (dependent) variable and X is the input (independent) variable.

Consider the following simple experiment in which we would like to measure reaction time for a group of individuals that are given *either* a drug or a placebo.[2] In this simple scenario, we have two variables: (i) the dependent variable (the outcome), which is the measure of reaction time, and (ii) the independent variable (the input), which is whether the individual in the group received a drug or a placebo. We consider this to be a simple experiment because it is not complex, even though it may seem complicated. Here, only one factor is used to influence a measured outcome.

In our simple experiment, we can control many elements that could have an influence on the outcome. In controlling these external influences, we are attempting to restrict the different forms of bias that will blur the real effects of our independent variable on the observed outcome. Bias can take many forms, so as we design our simple experiment, we think about the various biases that can occur, and we work to control these influences. For example, to reduce the likelihood of selection bias, we may randomly select our sample of experiment participants from a large population of diverse individuals. Next, rather than trying to get to know our sample of experiment

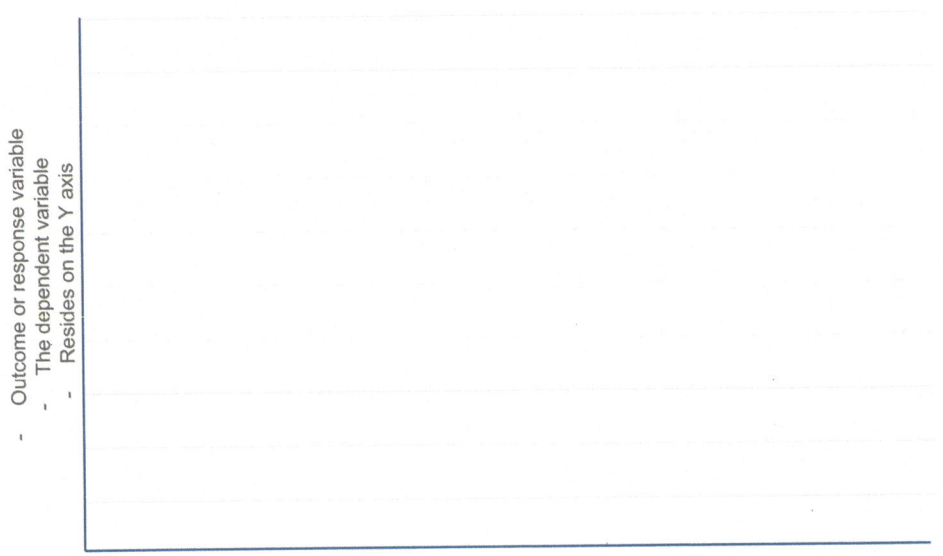

Figure 3.1 The dependent and independent variables.

participants, we randomly allocate these individuals to either the drug group (group 1) or the placebo group (group 2), as noted in Figure 3.2.

In Figure 3.3, the independent variable (presented on the X-axis – the horizontal axis) has two groups, and these groups are labelled either Group 1: the group receiving the drug or Group 2: the group receiving the placebo. Therefore, the data contained in the variable X (the independent variable) is at a nominal level of measurement and can have either of the following two values: drug or placebo. If we choose to process these data points mathematically, we could change the value of the drug to the numeral 1 and the value of placebo to the numeral 0.

In Figure 3.3, we see that the dependent variable (presented on the Y-axis – the vertical axis) is the measure of reaction time. Here, we stated the units of measurement; in this scenario we will choose to use reaction time measured in seconds. The values of the reaction time measurements are presented as decimal numerals ranging between 0 seconds to a maximum value of 1.00 second, but the level of measurement used to establish the precision of the reaction time observation is entirely up to the discretion of the experimenter.

After we have organized our two groups, administered the treatment (drug versus placebo), and measured the reaction times, then we process the data using an appropriate statistical methodology to determine if any observed difference in reaction times between the group receiving the drug is different than that of the group receiving the placebo. This final step is important to provide information about the drug effects on reaction time and therefore contributes to our development of knowledge on this specific topic. Likewise, during the analytical process, we can evaluate our initial hypothesis to determine the accuracy of our statement of expectation. During this analytical stage, we determine how much we can establish the generalizability of our experimental findings to a larger population of individuals not involved in our simple experiment.

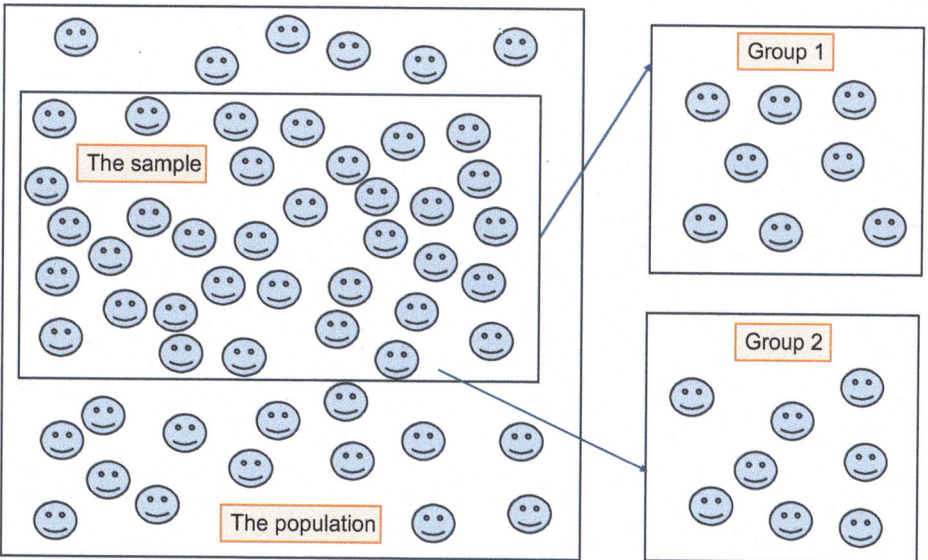

Figure 3.2 Random selection from a population and random allocation of participants from a sample to either of two groups.

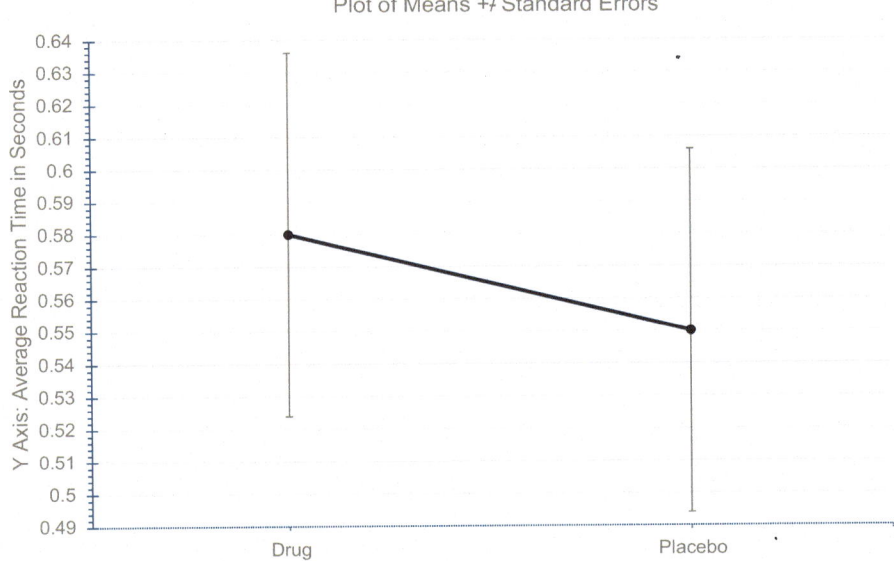

Figure 3.3 Graphical presentation of experiment outcomes.

The example of the experiment shown here represents a basic level of comparison. There are multiple ways that we could re-organize the design of our research question that would add to the complicated nature of what we are attempting to evaluate in the experimental design. For example, we could add additional independent variables, such as age or sex, upon which we could organize the data. We could also add different amounts of the drug supplied to the experiment participants as a subgroup within the Drug group.

In this example, we as researchers were able to control many elements of the experiment. For example, we decided from which population we would draw our sample of participants. Next, we decided how many participants we would randomly select from the original population. Then, we decided on the order by which we would randomly allocate the participants from the sample to each of the treatment groups (i.e., Drug or Placebo); and we decided how many participants we would allocate to either the Drug or Placebo group. After completing the data collection, we processed the data and determined the extent to which we can establish that by intervening with a drug, we were able to observe a reaction time that was different than that which occurred for a group of participants that consumed a placebo.

3.2 The Natural Experiment

There is, however, a type of experimental design in which the researcher can compare outcomes from two or more groups but in which they do not have control over the population, the sample, or the treatment variables. As noted by Humphreys et al. (2016), Craig et al. (2017), and Crane et al. (2020), the natural experiment is a form of research designed to compare two or more groups on an outcome measure for which the groups of individuals have self-selected to the different levels of the treatment, intervention, or suspected stimulus. That is, in the natural experiment, the groups form naturally and are not allocated by the investigator. Rather, in the natural experiment, the comparison groups and hence the individuals within the comparison groups are identified after the respective groups have formed. In addition, most often, the measure of interest or outcome variable is also determined and evaluated after the initial group formation has occurred.

Natural experiments emerge from real-world scenarios (Crane et al., 2020) and thus lack the randomization of participants to the different groups we might expect to observe in a formal, pre-planned, traditional experiment. Notwithstanding this limitation, natural experiments provide valuable opportunities for investigators to observe outcomes in groups which could not be organized beforehand because of various limitations, one such limitation being ethical concerns or considerations.

Consider an experiment in which an investigator wished to test the effects of a condition of interest such as, for example, an intervention, a stimulus, a treatment, or a substance that was known to have adverse health consequences on a group of individuals. While an experiment of this type may never be approved as a potential research investigation, the conditions of the comparison may already exist for a segment of society. That is, some individuals currently might be exposed to the condition of interest as part of their daily routine without considering the potential harm that exposure to such a condition could cause. Here, a natural experiment would be to identify the group of individuals that are exposed to the condition of interest as a result of their normal regimen and a group of individuals that have never used or been exposed to the condition of interest.

In this scenario, the investigator, after determining a sufficient number to represent the sample of members in the exposed and non-exposed groups, could then compare the effect of exposure to the known condition of interest on an outcome variable measured on all members of both groups. After investigating the characteristics of the exposed and non-exposed groups with respect to possible interactions with the condition of interest, any observed differences in the outcome measure between the two groups may then be attributed to the exposure to the condition of interest. In this way, the investigator can evaluate the observed outcome for the group of exposed individuals and compare the outcome against the measured response for the group of non-exposed individuals.

3.3 Dr. John Snow and a Historical Application of a Natural Experiment

Although there were many accounts of death (mortality) and illness (morbidity) throughout the centuries of discovery from the 1300s to the 1800s, the formalization of epidemic accounting was not common among healthcare providers. One of the early noted applications of epidemiological methods in public health was that used by Dr. John Snow in the mid-1800s when he investigated the relationship between the consumption of contaminated water and the incidence of death due to cholera. John Snow (1813–1858) was a physician who lived and worked in London, England. In addition to his reputation as an anaesthetist to Queen Victoria, he used the design of a natural experiment to demonstrate the causal association between the waterborne bacterium *Vibrio cholerae pucini 1854* (Tulchinsky, 2018) and the acute intestinal infection that led to death among citizens of London and, more specifically, the Soho district and residents that used the Broad Street pump between August and September 1854.

In the 1800s, houses in England did not have direct plumbing to provide running water, and so fresh water was supplied by water companies that established pumping stations in specific neighborhoods throughout England (Broich, 2007). In the larger cities like London, the water supply business was competitive during this era, and various companies competed for the rights to supply households with fresh water, most often drawn from the Thames River to areas of the City of London. Unfortunately, the Thames River was not only the source of fresh water, but it was also the natural sewer into which raw sewage from various neighborhoods flowed (Johnson, 2006).

During the 1830s, there were epidemics which spread across Europe, and although they were described as cholera, they were attributed to social unrest and political upheaval. A later widespread epidemic in 1848 led John Snow to publish a public health pamphlet that described the spread of cholera as being a waterborne infection. He suggested that the spread of cholera was indeed caused by drinking contaminated water rather than the commonly held belief that the illness was a result of bad air smells known as miasma. The miasma theory (also called the miasmatic theory) was a commonly accepted theory which considered that diseases and outbreaks like cholera or the bubonic plague and even sexually transmitted diseases like chlamydia were caused by a noxious form of "bad air," also known as night air (Johnson, 2006).

In 1854, the City of London experienced a major cholera outbreak, which many in positions of power (the judges, ministers, and lawmakers) believed to be caused by bad smells coming from the cesspools into which raw sewage flowed. However, Snow was a scientist, and he set out to prove that the theory of miasma was incorrect. Specifically, John Snow used the methodology of a natural experiment to ascertain that the cause of illness and death could be attributed to drinking water that was infested with the bacteria *Vibrio cholerae*. Considering that the different water companies sourced their water from various parts of the Thames River, Snow realized that some companies drew their water from areas upstream, where water was slightly cleaner, while others used downstream locations for their water supply – regions which were in the path of the flow of raw sewage.

Snow used the approach of a natural experiment to compare a cohort of ill individuals and a control group of individuals that did not demonstrate similar illness. In this scenario, the natural experiment considered the prevalence of cholera as an outcome resulting from naturally occurring events not influenced by the investigator. Here, Snow identified individuals from the same general municipal area that were customers of two separate water companies which competed in supplying water to the neighborhoods. Snow chose the Lambeth water company as one of the suppliers, knowing that it had moved its intake spout upstream following a previous suggestion that they were the cause of an earlier cholera outbreak, and the Southwark and Vauxhall Company as the other water supplier, which had an intake spout downstream from the effluent discharge. Snow's hypothesis was that the customers who consumed water supplied by the Southwark and Vauxhall Company were more likely to present with cholera and cholera-like symptoms because of exposure to the causal agent (*Vibrio cholerae*) present in water downstream of the effluent discharge spout than persons in households that received their water from the Lambeth Water Company, which drew its water from above the effluent discharge spout.

In the natural experiment, once the two groups are identified, the researcher monitors the individuals within the two groups and records the outcomes. Snow monitored customers from each water company by visiting the households and simply counting and comparing the number of cases of cholera in each group of patrons. In other words, he let the events occur naturally and without his direct influence on the stimulus or the outcome (Tulchinsky, 2018).

In Snow's recounting of deaths from the designated areas within the time period of his study, he noted that 330 of 334 total deaths could be attributed to water consumption – most notably the presence of the bacteria *Vibrio cholerae*. His data showed that in comparing cases of death between the two water companies within the Soho neighborhood, patrons from the Southwark and Vauxhall company that were supplied water from the Broad Street pump showed a higher incidence of death from cholera. Deaths among Southwark and Vauxhall company customers were 286 compared to only 14 deaths among patrons of the Lambeth water company.

In addition, Snow compared his findings among customers of the water companies against other nearby locations to contrast the number of attributable deaths. For example, down the street from the Broad Street pump was the Broad Street brewery, where some 70 workers were given an allowance of free beer every day. No cholera-associated fatalities were recorded among brewery workers during the time period that Snow had selected. Likewise, in a review of the 530 inmates of the Poland Street workhouse, which was around the corner from the Broad Street pump, only five individuals had contracted cholera; but since the workhouse had its own well, none of the inmates drank from the Broad Street water source.

For his part, John Snow removed the pump handle from the Broad Street Pump, requiring patrons to draw their water from other sources, which subsequently led to a drop in cholera-related deaths and thereby supported his hypothesis that it was indeed the Southwark and Vauxhall Water supply that caused the cholera outbreak. Snow's diligent observations confirmed that patrons of the Southwark and Vauxhall Water Company were eight times more likely to die from cholera than patrons of the Lambeth Water Company. Furthermore, by applying the natural experiment methodology, Snow was able to advance the current level of knowledge about germ theory over the commonly held belief that breathing "stinky air" as purported by the miasmatic theory was the cause of various infectious diseases (Johnson, 2006).

In a 2017 position paper, the World Health Organization[3] described cholera as an acute intestinal infection that is caused by the *Vibrio cholerae* bacterium and causes individuals to experience severe diarrhoea, leading to dehydration and eventually death. One of the ways the infection is treated is by rehydration through copious consumption of clean water. However, most often, the difficulty is the ability to locate clean water that could flush the *Vibrio cholerae* from the individual!

3.4 The Epidemiological Triad

Although epidemiological applications have evolved beyond the study of infectious diseases and the need to provide proof for germ theory, often in the epidemiological process, practitioners assess determinants of health or probable causes of disease while considering the host, the agent, and the environment. Together, these three constructs comprise the epidemiologic triad (Méndez-Martínez et al., 2018; Jia et al., 2020).

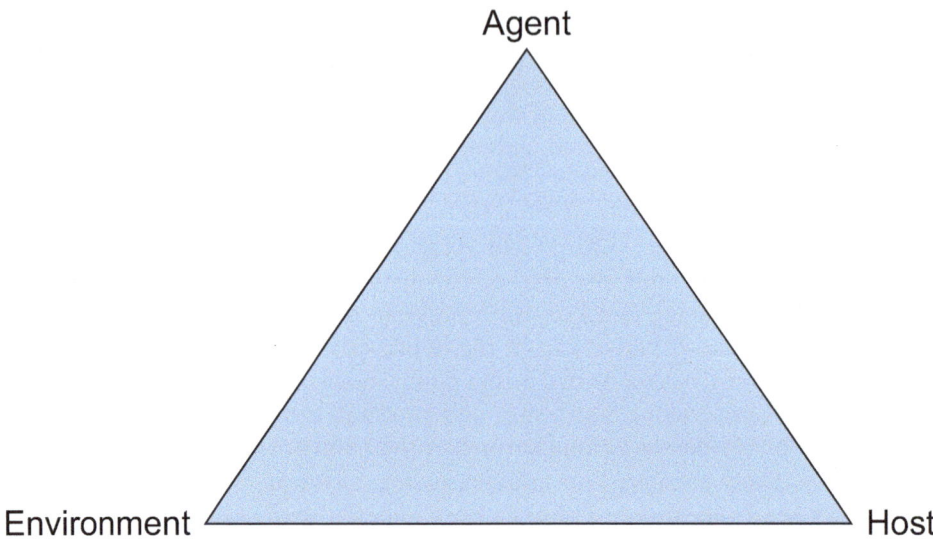

Figure 3.4 The epidemiological triad.

Beginning with the suspected causal agent, the epidemiological triad exists when an external agent, typically a suspected causal stimulus, is present and has been purported to initiate a measurable outcome to occur. Given that epidemiological applications are now accepted widely in practices beyond studies of infectious disease, the designation of agent has also broadened to include many suspected causal mechanisms such as chemical contaminants, physical forces, and hereditable pathways that lead to intergenerational diseases and conditions, to name only a few examples. While it is recognized that an agent must exist to form the epidemiological triad, the presence of an identifiable agent alone is not always sufficient to cause disease. Despite our best investigative methods, we realize that a variety of factors influence whether exposure to an organism will result in disease, including the organism's pathogenicity (ability to cause disease), as well as the volume of exposure – the dose.

Yet disease processes are only one aspect of epidemiological applications for the triad. As noted by Magarey and Trexler (2020), adding the provision of information, not as a noun but as a verb (*v. to provide information*), to the epidemiological triad can expand its functionality, especially in the application of the triad to understanding dynamics of events in social epidemiology and the spread of harmful, inaccurate, and intentionally untrue information. Understanding the influence of information, or more importantly, misinformation, as an agent at the vertex[4] is critical to understanding its effect as an influence on the host in the environment of social epidemics.

The host is the next vertex of the epidemiological triad. The host refers to the individual that can develop or contract the disease. Several risk factors underlie the susceptibility of a host to be affected by the agent (or causal mechanism). In measuring health outcomes, behaviors and personal choices are often important influencing factors. However, the susceptibility of an individual (the host) to be affected by the agent can include many predisposing factors. An emerging example is conditions that affect one's DNA, either directly – causing deletions and mutations to the DNA sequence – or indirectly as those we observe in the transient effect of methylation, whereby the activity of the DNA segment is influenced but without a change to the DNA sequence.

The third vertex in the epidemiological triad is the environment. The environment represents those opportunistic conditions that enable the increased likelihood that the condition will be present and measurable. The environment can describe the extrinsic factors that affect the agent and the opportunity for exposure. In the grand scheme, the environment can be the biosphere! It can include physical factors such as geology and climate, biologic factors such as insects that transmit the agent (the causal mechanism), and socioeconomic factors such as crowding, sanitation, and the availability – or lack thereof – of health services.

3.5 Epidemiology as a Modus Operandi

Epidemiology provides the tools for us to understand the wicked problems we encounter when trying to make sense of health. While communicable (infectious) diseases catch our attention because they are difficult to predict, have rapid population impacts and uncontrolled spread, non-communicable diseases (Patel and Webster, 2016), adverse social conditions – poverty and racial injustice (Parolin and Lee, 2022; Gweshengwe and Hassan, 2020) – and environmental crises quietly but progressively reached global pandemic proportions and, as such, were laid bare because of COVID-19 (Tanveer et al., 2020).

Gathering data for epidemiological processes specifically designed to address health issues is invaluable in providing essential information about emerging health concerns at various levels of the population. Without question, there is an urgent need to increase our collection of evidence to support decisions by policymakers and program planners. The value of integrating information collected from sampling biophysical and socioeconomic data resources to establish relationships across health conditions cannot be understated. However, the methods by which we collect these data to supply our information repositories remain complicated.

According to Thacker et al. (1989), epidemiological surveillance methods which are based on a systematic collection of data can assist us in collecting, analyzing and interpreting health data. Managing health data from surveillance systems can provide essential information to health policymakers and program planners in the development and implementation stages of interventions and community campaigns as well as during the evaluation. Health data, collected through surveillance or direct monitoring, along with the processes of data mining, can help us to recognize unusual events such as outbreaks of disease (e.g., cholera, Ebola, SARS, COVID-19) or emerging health issues as we see in studies of the climate crisis (glacial melting, coastal erosion, wildfire prevalence), and social inequality in the form of poverty, unemployment, and racial injustice.

The term *surveillance* is derived from the French *sur* – over – and *veiller* – to watch (Choi, 2018). To conduct surveillance requires us to maintain a continuous observation of a cohort, community, or population. In public health, surveillance was described by Declich and Carter (1994) to be the system that provides an ongoing collection of health data. In a more recent explanation of public health surveillance systems by Groseclose and Buckeridge (2017), the authors described the process as not only collecting data but also evaluating the quality of the data, managing the data for analyses, and interpreting the results to provide knowledge translation and dissemination of information. Applied in this way, the processes of surveillance are not unidimensional but are multidimensional and can provide valuable information for the evaluation of public health issues of concern.

According to Arita et al. (2004) and Hong et al. (2020), surveillance systems are valuable resources for identifying risks to public health by monitoring events and behaviors at the community and population levels. Established surveillance methods within a community can supply comprehensive and timely accounts of risk factors that underlie potential adverse public health events. The information supplied through regular monitoring of the surveillance systems can be used to prepare event mitigation strategies that can include but are not limited to education programs designed to inform the public about risk factor prevention, promotion of positive health behaviors, and various interventions that focus directly on the public health event or that address the risk factors of the event.

Prior to 2020, surveillance systems followed a variety of approaches that included passive systems (Hong et al., 2020) and active systems (Deckert et al., 2021), which included derivatives of each system such as the sentinel-based systems (Arita et al., 2004). Regardless of whether the surveillance system was active or passive, each used a specific and clearly defined approach to data collection and monitoring of potential public health events.

The passive surveillance system is defined as a process that uses existing personnel in healthcare systems to collect routine data following a chronological schedule or as the data emerges (Murray and Cohen, 2017; Hong et al., 2020). While passive surveillance systems can uncover trends in the identification of diseases and conditions through standardized reporting, a limitation of the passive surveillance system, as noted by Hong and coworkers, is that although the system has a low overhead and is generally inexpensive, it may have issues establishing or maintaining quality in the process of data reporting. Notifiable disease reporting is an example of passive surveillance in that it requires individuals to report on very specific diseases when the cases emerge within a cohort or community (Murray and Cohen, 2017).

Active surveillance systems described by Deckert et al. (2021) are based on routine testing for risk factors and continuous monitoring of events which help to identify and then isolate individuals that are determined to be case positive despite their reported symptoms. Implementation of active surveillance methods enables rapid responses to public health events which may be emerging and thereby prevents further spread – as in the application to infectious disease monitoring or event mitigation – as in responses to public health disasters.

By using an active surveillance approach, health officials can determine incidence rates (the number of new cases within a given time period) as well as prevalence rates (the total number of cases for all those at risk), which provide important information to support action.

The typical sentinel-based surveillance system (Arita et al., 2004; Guillot et al., 2022) can be described as a type of active surveillance system because it is purposeful and deliberate in collecting specific data from designated sites within a fixed network. For example, a network of healthcare settings may be designated as data-reporting nodes within a planned area. In the sentinel surveillance approach, the data will be collected by individuals which can include, for example, healthcare providers, laboratory technicians, and volunteers. By situating data-collection nodes in various regions that are suspected to have a known distribution of a disease or condition of interest, the sentinel surveillance system can capture data from a larger geographic area using strategically placed data-collection sites (Guillot et al., 2022). Yet one limitation of the sentinel surveillance approach is that it is fixed to a specific network that may restrict observations to only those occurring in the network and thereby miss events that occur outside the catchment areas of the sentinel sites.

Given that active surveillance strategies are most often used in emergency situations, as in disease outbreaks where the disease is targeted for eradication or elimination, and where every case must be found and investigated, when the World Health Organization declared COVID-19 to be a pandemic as of March 11, 2020, most (but not all) countries of the world enacted some form of active surveillance strategy, whether it was a traditional approach or a new, modified system derived from a combination of systems.

A recent report by Liu et al. (2023) described the sentinel community-based surveillance system as an active approach to collecting essential data to build critical information for rapid responses to important health concerns. As noted by Liu and colleagues, since the COVID-19 pandemic, surveillance approaches have shifted from passive to active approaches that provide essential information in a timely (explicitly scheduled) and accurate manner. In addition, the surveillance approaches are transitioning away from "patient-centered" sampling, which tends to focus on specific disease conditions, to "people-centered" samples, which focus on the general population and are therefore more inclusive in capturing multiple conditions (Liu et al., 2023).

According to Liu and coworkers, the sentinel community-based surveillance system considers the entire life cycle of disease management that includes (i) prevention, (ii) screening, (iii) diagnosis, (iv) treatment, (v) rehabilitation, and (vi) social supports. By integrating these attributes into the administrative records that include medical care and social care, Liu suggested that they had formed a complete and comprehensive system that can accommodate the necessary data collection, data processing for knowledge creation, and knowledge translation that is essential in controlling the spread of future infectious diseases.

3.6 Fundamental Concepts of Association and Causation

In many applications of epidemiological methods, rather than observing cause-and-effect relationships, we observe relationships between variables that represent exposures and outcomes. Thus, in applying epidemiological methods, we are cautious to consider that any seemingly apparent association between an exposure and an outcome could have resulted from an alternative explanation. Hence the reason John Snow included the record of deaths from the Broad Street brewery and the Polland Street workhouse in his evidence that the suspected source of *Vibrio cholerae* was specifically from the Southwark and Vauxhall water company.

Associations have statistical implications because they refer to the dependence between at least two variables representing measured outcomes. Associations may describe clusters of responses among cohorts of individuals, or they can demonstrate the consistency of responses for two or more measurements for a given individual. However, although associations help us to understand many elements of relationships in the data that we collect through epidemiological approaches, the use of associations to demonstrate causation is highly specific (Lucas and McMichael, 2005).

Causation is a fundamental concept of epidemiology (Parascandola and Weed, 2001) and can be described within the epidemiological triad (Jia et al., 2019). For example, we say causation represents a logical series of events that begin with a condition, that is a stimulus or a characteristic, as in an agent, that, when introduced to an individual or cohort, as in a sample or even a population – the host – within a given environment produces a measurable outcome. Most often, causation is measured in relation to an outcome like illness, injury, disease state, or health status. In epidemiological applications, we infer causation based on associations with selected factors that have been externally validated as causal mechanisms. The limitation in epidemiological inference based on an association between a factor and an outcome is that while exposure to a factor might cause a specific outcome, we can only suggest that the suspected causal mechanism is, at best, a risk factor for the condition of interest. This builds on the recommendation that no single study is sufficient for causal inference, and this is especially true for observational (epidemiological) investigations. However, the importance of associations in establishing causation is bolstered by the premise that an association is considered more likely to be causal when it is demonstrated in multiple circumstances and especially when the circumstances are based on different populations, different scenarios, and different applications. Under such circumstances, strong associations are less likely to be explained by chance or bias.

In 1965, Sir Bradford Hill established nine criteria for determining causation based on observed associations (Fedak et al., 2015; Giancolo et al., 2020). Hill's Criteria for Causality are presented in Table 3.1. Despite that all of these criteria have been extensively debated within the scientific community, they provide a simple checklist approach (Lucas and McMichael, 2005) for assessing the importance of associations as risk factors to determine causal mechanisms.

Beginning with the strength of association, Hill suggested this was self-evident in the data accumulated in many epidemiological applications. For example, Hill drew upon the evidence that death rates among cigarette smokers were nine to ten times higher than among non-smokers and that heavy smokers were twenty to thirty times more likely to die prematurely than non-smokers. While this evidence may seem overwhelmingly simple to understand – and it certainly begs the question, why didn't we stop smoking in 1965 when Hill made these remarks? – the strength of association alone may not provide sufficient information to counter the contrarians' argument.

Table 3.1 Hill's Criteria for Causation[5]

1	Strength of the association
2	Consistency of the observed association
3	Specificity of the observed association
4	Temporality of the observed association – the importance of the sequence of events
5	The measure of a biological gradient – as in a dose–response relationship
6	Biological plausibility
7	Coherence – the presence of other supporting evidence
8	Experimental evidence (or quasi-experimental evidence – as in the natural experiments)
9	Analogy – demonstrations by other events

Often, additional evidence is required to eliminate suspected confounding associations, and there is a need to provide proof to support what may seem obvious even when the strength of the association is less than profound.

Hill next suggested the criteria of consistency, which he described as being able to demonstrate repeatability of an outcome by different persons, places, and times and for different circumstances. Yet Hill also cautioned that the randomness of these events may lead some to suggest that the observation may not overcome the observation occurring by chance. In this regard, statistical probability may restrict acceptance of a possible outcome.

The criterion of consistency is followed by the criterion of specificity. Here, Hill drew a relationship between time, place, and person – three essential characteristics of causal factors. If the environment were such that it could be considered a predisposing factor for an outcome, and the only reason that a person was identified as having the condition of interest was because they were exposed to the environment while comparators were not exposed, then the specificity of the suggested causal mechanism could be supported. For example, if the condition of interest was lung cancer and the person smoked, compared to an individual who did not have lung cancer and did not smoke, the condition of specificity would be supported. However, specificity alone does not infer causation, and this apparent association can surely be enumerated by arranging the comparison of cohort outcomes as shown in Figure 3.5, for example.

In Figure 3.5, we observe the arrangement of conditions leading to cases and non-cases of lung cancer for smokers versus non-smokers. This 2 × 2 or fourfold table is

	+ lung cancer	- lung cancer
Smoker	(A) Smoked and was diagnosed with lung cancer	(B) Smoked but was not diagnosed with lung cancer
Non-smoker	(C) Never smoked but was diagnosed with lung cancer	(D) Never smoked and was not diagnosed with lung cancer

Figure 3.5 Arrangement of the data to calculate specificity.

used to calculate the specificity estimate associated with developing lung cancer. In the arrangement of the data, we are not only considering those individuals that smoked and developed lung cancer (Cell A) against those individuals that never smoked and as expected did not develop cancer (Cell D), but in using this 2 × 2 arrangement, we are also able to adjust the calculation to account for those individuals that never smoked but developed lung cancer (Cell C), as well as for those individuals that smoked but never developed lung cancer (Cell B). The calculation of specificity is given as a percentage and is based on the number of cases recorded in Cell D divided by the sum of cases in Cell B plus Cell D, arranged as shown in Equation 3.1 (Trevethan, 2017).

EQUATION 3.1 CALCULATION OF SPECIFICITY FROM A FOURFOLD TABLE

$$\text{Specificity} = (\text{Cell D} \div (\text{Cell B} + \text{Cell D})) \times 100$$

As noted by Fedak et al. (2015), the criterion of temporality is the most useful of Hill's criteria because it states that the horse must come before the cart. That is, we need to have exposure to the causal mechanism before we can expect to observe the condition of interest. Establishing a biological gradient – as in a dose–response relationship, was Hill's fifth criteria, and although it suggests a linear relationship between the volume of exposure and outcome, we can expect that there are variants to this relationship which continue to support the basic notion – as we increase exposure to a suspected causal factor, despite that it may be non-linear, we increase the risk of demonstrating the condition of interest.

Confirming biological plausibility was the sixth criterion suggested by Hill, meaning that there was sufficient underlying knowledge about the association between a suspected cause and corresponding outcome to consider the mechanism viable. However, even Hill pointed out that such criteria were fraught with folly as we continue to develop new knowledge and therefore should not discount an association because we do not know better.

The criterion of coherence – the seventh criterion – is a companion to the criterion of biological plausibility (number 6) and suggests that we regard the evidence as valuable. Our current ability to use high-throughput analysis (Fadak et al., 2015) enables us to gather evidence quickly and comprehensively so that we can evaluate extremely complex hypotheses in a noticeably brief period. This ability is imperative to decision-making regarding accepting or rejecting suggested associations between suspected causal factors and observed outcomes.

Experimental evidence, as suggested by criterion eight, is important, as noted by Hill (1965), but as Fedak et al. stated, the complexity of research questions is as important in gathering essential data to support the presence of a suspected causal mechanism. Finally, the ninth criteria was analogy, which Hill suggested may be the evidence needed to accept a relationship between a suspected causal mechanism and an observed outcome if the suspected causal mechanism was implicated in other similar relationships with other conditions.

As scientific methods have evolved over the past 50 years, so has our ability to build statistical models of association. While this may lead many to question the salient nature of Hill's classic criteria, it does not discount the importance of these criteria as an intuitive first step in considering *causal* mechanisms of health outcomes.

3.6.1 Discussion Questions

1   In this chapter, we noted that by providing timely access to high-quality relevant information about trends and behaviors at a population level, and by establishing systems of health surveillance and tools to measure health service compliance and data from diagnostic outcomes, practitioners, researchers, and policymakers can make informed decisions that impact the health of populations, communities, and ultimately individuals. How were the considerations of epidemiology used in dealing with the COVID-19 pandemic? What were some of the barriers and challenges that health specialists faced in operationalizing epidemiological methods during the pandemic?

2   The criteria for causation were included in this chapter. Consider an application of the criteria for causation for a real-world health issue – not the pandemic but perhaps a potential outbreak of another condition or disease. How does each step of the criteria relate to your condition of interest?

Notes

1   According to the World Health Organization, the virus that caused the coronavirus 19 disease was named severe acute respiratory syndrome coronavirus 2 (SARS-CoV-2). Retrieved from: Naming the coronavirus disease (COVID-19) and the virus that causes it (who.int).

2   A placebo is simply defined as a control agent. In a drug study, the placebo has all of the physical characteristics of the drug but without the active ingredient of the drug.

3   Summary Cholera 2017 World Health Organization – retrieved 02/25/2021 www.who.int/immunization/policy/position_papers/PP_Cholera_2017_summary.pdf.

4   The term *vertex* refers to the corner angle. Here, it is one of the corners in a triangular shape of the epidemiological triad.

5   From Hill's Presidential Address in the Proceedings of the Royal Society of Medicine, January 14, 1965.

References

Arita I, Nakane M, Kojima K, Yoshihara N, Nakano T, El-Gohary A. Role of a sentinel surveillance system in the context of global surveillance of infectious diseases [published correction appears in Lancet Infect Dis. 2004 Aug;4(8):533]. *Lancet Infect Dis.* 2004;4(3):171–177. doi:10.1016/S1473-3099(04)00942-9

Broich J. Engineering the empire: British water supply systems and colonial societies, 1850–1900. *J Br Stud.* 2007;46(2):346–365. doi:10.1086/510891 (Accessed 30 August 2023).

Choi BC. The past, present, and future of public health surveillance [published correction appears in Scientifica (Cairo). 2018 Jul 2;2018:6943062]. *Scientifica (Cairo).* 2012;2012:875253. doi:10.6064/2012/875253/

Craig P, Katikireddi SV, Leyland A, Popham F. Natural experiments: An overview of methods, approaches, and contributions to public health intervention research. *Annu Rev Public Health.* 2017;38:39–56. doi:10.1146/annurev-publhealth-031816-044327

Crane M, Bohn-Goldbaum E, Grunseit A, Bauman A. Using natural experiments to improve public health evidence: A review of context and utility for obesity prevention. *Health Res Policy Sys* 2020;18:48. doi:10.1186/s12961-020-00564-2

Deckert A, Anders S, de Allegri M, et al. Effectiveness and cost-effectiveness of four different strategies for SARS-CoV-2 surveillance in the general population (CoV-Surv Study): A structured summary of a study protocol for a cluster-randomised, two-factorial controlled trial. *Trials.* 2021;22(1):39. doi:10.1186/s13063-020-04982-z

Declich S, Carter AO. Public health surveillance: Historical origins, methods and evaluation. *Bull World Health Organ.* 1994;72(2):285–304.

Fedak KM, Bernal A, Capshaw ZA, Gross S. Applying the Bradford Hill criteria in the 21st century: How data integration has changed causal inference in molecular epidemiology. *Emerg Themes Epidemiol.* 2015;12:14. doi:10.1186/s12982-015-0037-4

Fox MP, Murray EJ, Lesko CR, Sealy-Jefferson S. On the need to revitalize descriptive epidemiology. *Am J Epidemiol.* 2022;191(7):1174–1179. doi:10.1093/aje/kwac056

Gianicolo EAL, Eichler M, Muensterer O, Strauch K, Blettner M. Methods for evaluating causality in observational studies. *Dtsch Arztebl Int.* 2020;116(7):101–107. doi:10.3238/arztebl.2020.0101

Groseclose SL, Buckeridge DL. Public health surveillance systems: Recent advances in their use and evaluation. *Ann Rev Public Health.* 2017;38(1):57–79.

Guillot C, Bouchard C, Aenishaenslin C, Berthiaume P, Milord F, Leighton PA. Criteria for selecting sentinel unit locations in a surveillance system for vector-borne disease: A decision tool. *Front Public Health.* 2022;10:1003949. doi:10.3389/fpubh.2022.1003949

Gweshengwe B, Hassan NH. Defining the characteristics of poverty and their implications for poverty analysis. *Cogent Soc Sci.* 2020;6:1. doi:10.1080/23311886.2020.1768669

Hill AB. The environment and disease: Association or causation? *J Royal Soc Med.* 1965;58:295–300.

Hong R, Walker R, Hovan G, Henry L, Pescatore R. The power of public health surveillance. *Dela J Public Health.* 2020;6(2):60–63. doi:10.32481/djph.2020.07.016

Humphreys DK, Panter J, Sahlqvist S, et al. Changing the environment to improve population health: A framework for considering exposure in natural experimental studies. *J Epidemiol Community Health.* 2016;70:941–946.

Jia P, Dong W, Yang S, Zhan Z, Tu L, Lai S. Spatial lifecourse epidemiology and infectious disease research. *Trends Parasitol.* 2020;36(3):235–238. doi:10.1016/j.pt.2019.12.012

Johnson S. *The Ghost Map.* Riverhead Books, New York, 2006, 299 pp.

Liu J, Li Q, Liang W, Liu M. Sentinel community-based surveillance: An innovative mode of proactive surveillance on infectious disease. *China CDC Wkly.* 2023;5(23):516–518. doi:10.46234/ccdcw2023.097

Lucas RM, McMichael AJ. Association or causation: Evaluating links between "environment and disease". *Bull World Health Organ.* 2005;83(10):792–795.

Magarey RD, Trexler CM. Information: A missing component in understanding and mitigating social epidemics. *Humanit Soc Sci Commun.* 2020;7:128. doi:10.1057/s41599-020-00620-w

Méndez-Martínez S, García-Carrasco M, Jiménez-Herrera EA, et al. Factors of the epidemiological triad that influence the persistence of human papilloma virus infection in women with systemic lupus erythematosus. *Lupus.* 2018;27(9):1542–1546. doi:10.1177/0961203318773176

Murray J, Cohen AL. Infectious disease surveillance. *Int Encyclop Pub Health.* 2017;222–229. doi:10.1016/B978-0-12-803678-5.00517-8

Osterholm MT, Hedberg CW. Epidemiologic principles. In *Mandell, Douglas, and Bennett's Principles and Practice of Infectious Diseases.* 2015:146–157.e2. doi:10.1016/B978-1-4557-4801-3.00013-8

Parascandola M, Weed DL. Causation in epidemiology. *J Epidemiol Commun Health.* 2001;55(12):905–912. doi:10.1136/jech.55.12.905

Parolin Z, Lee E. The role of poverty and racial discrimination in exacerbating the health consequences of COVID-19. *Lancet Reg Health Am.* 2022;7(3):1–8. doi:10.1016/j.lana.2021.100178

Patel A, Webster R. The potential and value of epidemiology in curbing non-communicable diseases. *Glob Health Epidemiol Genom.* 2016;1:e15. doi:10.1017/gheg.2016.10

Tanveer F, Khalil AT, Ali M, Shinwari ZK. Ethics, pandemic and environment; looking at the future of low middle income countries. *Int J Equity Health*. 2020;19(1):182. doi:10.1186/s12939-020-01296-z

Thacker SB, Parrish RG, Trowbridge FL. A method for evaluating systems of epidemiological surveillance. *World Health Stat Q*. 1988;41(1):11–8. Erratum in: World Health Stat Q 1989;42(2): preceding 58.

Trevethan R. Sensitivity, specificity, and predictive values: Foundations, liabilities, and pitfalls in research and practice. *Front Public Health*. 2017;5:307. doi:10.3389/fpubh.2017.00307

Tulchinsky TH. John Snow, cholera, the broad street pump; waterborne diseases then and now. *Case Stud Pub Health*. 2018:77–99. doi:10.1016/B978-0-12-804571-8.00017-2

Udell JA, Behrouzi B, Sivaswamy A, et al. Clinical risk, sociodemographic factors, and SARS-CoV-2 infection over time in Ontario, Canada. *Sci Rep*. 2022;12(1):1–14. doi:10.1038/s41598-022-13598-z

Wachtler B, Michalski N, Nowossadeck E, et al. Socioeconomic inequalities and COVID-19 – a review of the current international literature. *J Health Monit*. 2020;5(Suppl 7):3–17. doi:10.25646/7059

CHAPTER 4

The Social Determinants of Health

4.0 Introduction

The World Health Organization (WHO) defines social determinants of health (SDOH) as conditions or circumstances in which people are born, grow, live, work, and age (World Health Organization, 2008). These conditions are influenced by many different social, political, and economic factors, and in turn, these factors have both direct and indirect influences on our health and well-being. As such, the health of the population depends on a socio-politico-economic framework that provides adequate social resources for all and promotes equitable distribution of resources across citizens. The quality, quantity, and dispersal of social resources, which includes educational opportunities, along with adequate employment, healthcare, access to nutritious foods, healthy and culturally safe environments, and neighborhoods/communities where violence and risk of personal injury are minimized, largely determine the health of the individual and the community.

4.1 Well-Being, Salutogenesis, and the Social Determinants of Health

The terms *health*, *well-being*, *salutogenesis*, and the *determinants of health* have been explained, defined, and described throughout health research literature. As a result, there are many examples of these terms used by researchers, educators, and policymakers to support various approaches that purport to realize higher states of personal fulfillment for the human species. Whereas we noted in Chapter 1 of this text that the term *health* has multiple definitions and considerations, the term *well-being* is equally as interchangeable and is often used with literary license to describe an inherently positive perspective (Simons and Baldwin, 2021).

The term *well-being* is neither unique nor novel in defining or contextualizing health. Rather, as noted by Jarden and Roache (2023), the concept of well-being has been pondered for thousands of years. At its core, well-being is accepted as multidimensional and based on subjective dimensions that represent feelings or perceived positive

DOI: 10.4324/9781003474777-4

emotions which can include, for example, happiness and satisfaction. Hence, the term *well-being* often includes the disclaimer "subjective" in describing one's perception of well-being since it represents a value judgement of a person's state of being. Clearly, the challenge in describing well-being is a result of the multiplicity of ways that well-being is both measured and reported in the literature. For example, Bautista and coworkers (2023), reported that the term *well-being* has been used to represent constructs such as quality of life, wellness, or happiness as unique outcome estimates of a person's perceived state. Similarly, the term *well-being* has been used to represent a conglomerate of variables that, when combined and evaluated, are used to describe an individual's subjective well-being as a latent variable.[1] The most recent World Health Organization definition for well-being (WHO, 2021) is intentional in describing well-being as a positive state for individuals as well as communities and, in so doing, describes not only its function – as a resource for daily life, but also the factors that determine its outcome with reference to social, economic, and environmental conditions.

Salutogenesis is a term coined by Anton Antonovsky (Mittelmark et al., 2022) as a perceived state within oneself that describes their recognition of the stresses of life and their ability to cope with such stresses. The salutogenic construct is based on the notion that individuals develop, from infancy, a *sense of coherence*, which can be described as a sense of recognizing and coping with the stimuli that make up one's internal and external environments. In creating the theory of salutogenesis, Antonovsky suggested a model in which salutogenesis emerges as a multifactorial construct that is shaped by the events within a human's development. These events include but are not limited to experiencing life events and the interaction of such life events on an individual's recognition of physical and mental strengths as well as their perception of self within their social order and their sense of having an ability to manage the feelings that arise from processing the complexity of input stimuli. Hence, salutogenesis is a sense of coherence (Mittlemark et al., 2017).

As noted by Raphael et al. (2019), the social determinants of health help to explain health outcomes and health inequities that lead to chronic disease and premature death through measurable conditions within societies. Some experts argue that the social determinants of health conjure two distinct meanings, referring either to (1) the factors that promote or detract from the health of the individual and of society, or (2) the policies and processes that lead to inequitable distribution of these resources across groups occupying different social tiers (Graham, 2004). For this chapter, we will use a comprehensive definition of the social determinants of health and consider all factors, policies, and processes that explain how our living and working conditions affect health and contribute to health inequities.

Measuring the extent to which the social determinants of health are recognized as important lays bare the inequity within a society and calls into question the social justice therein. Enhancing a society's capability to achieve a positive state of health can only occur when we recognize and act on social inequities related to health in terms of access, quality, and distribution of pertinent resources.

To optimize the potential for individuals and society to achieve positive states of health, we need to focus on the interrelatedness of social, environmental, and economic factors in our daily lives and in the lives of others. Here, we will explore the determinants of health. That is, we will consider those factors that influence the health of a population.

4.2 So, What Is a Determinant?

In the mathematics of linear algebra, a determinant is a factor that fixes an outcome. However, health is not mathematics. In health, we also have determinants, and although well accepted as a list of valid factors, such factors are not fixed. In health, the determinants are less precise, and often, they describe broad categories of living conditions that shape the quality of life that we experience daily.

The determinants of health are interactive, and each determinant's effect depends on the presence and strength of risk factors and protective factors. Further, as we will see, the relative contribution of those characteristics which we have labelled as the social determinants of health, abbreviated as SDOH, will vary across settings and groups. In this way, studying the singular contribution of individual determinants of health may be less meaningful than understanding their cumulative or interactive effects. What is more, the precise constellation and contribution of determinants depends on the specific health outcome of interest. As shown throughout health-related research, exploring the effects of the social determinants of health has fostered interest in understanding the interaction between the social determinants of health and associations with specific conditions, such as depression, oral health, and cardiovascular disease (Islam, 2019).

Table 4.1 provides a version of a list of social determinants of health. Although the list is extensive, it is not exhaustive. Other examples of determinants that have been documented in the literature, albeit less frequently, include media, internet access, and availability of time, whereby time is viewed as a determinant in that accessing health services, exercising, and engaging in other pro-health behaviors all require a time commitment. It is also important to note that depending on whether the focus is on predicting positive states of health or explaining health inequities across groups, different terminology may be used. For instance, researchers may study constructs of racism

Table 4.1 The Social Determinants of Health

1	Income and income distribution
2	Early childhood development
3	Employment and job security
4	Education and literacy
5	Personal health practices and coping skills
6	Food security
7	Neighborhood features (e.g., recreational opportunities; crime rates)
8	Social inclusion
9	Social safety net (e.g. social positioning or social status)
10	Housing
11	Health services
12	Geography
13	Gender and gender identity
14	Sexual orientation
15	Indigenous ancestry/Aboriginal Status
16	Immigration
17	Disability
18	Race and racism
19	Culture
20	Globalization

and discrimination in trying to explain inequitable outcomes across ethnic groups or may describe freedom from discrimination and violence as a requisite for good health. Likewise, social inclusion may be studied as a predictor of good health and as a buffer against risk factors, while social exclusion or isolation is framed as a barrier to good health or as an explanatory factor in describing health inequities.

In the U.S. Department of Health and Human Services' Healthy People 2030 agenda, the social determinants of health were organized into five domains: economics, education and literacy, access to healthcare, the environment, and the community. Social determinants can also be categorized as micro-level or macro-level variables depending on whether they refer to individual or interpersonal aspects of health or target structural or group-level factors and processes. In exploring the social determinants of health listed in Table 4.1, we consider how addressing these factors will improve health outcomes, not only for individuals but also for society, and how we might overcome health inequities that are associated with these factors.

Traditional efforts to address health inequities have focused on access to medical care. However, even in countries with universal access to healthcare, there remain large discrepancies in health outcomes reflective of social class. Biomedical models of health emphasize the accountability of the individual in pursuing health behaviors, like nutritious eating, regular physical activity, and maintaining healthcare appointments. A social-determinants-of-health perspective forces us to acknowledge that individuals exist in societies and that many of our health-related behaviors have social roots.

Creating an understanding and subsequent application of the social determinants of health as a mitigating framework that could guide societal change has led to the use of various models and metaphors to help explain their importance. A comprehensive model developed by Thimm-Kaiser et al. (2023) includes categorizing the social determinants of health in regard to their influence on person-centered activities – the micro level; social or group behavior changes which are considered to be the meso-level (Rhodes et al., 2004); and schemes that are instituted by policymakers within government or the macro-level.

Together, these categories support a heuristic – a decision-making strategy that uses limited information (Marewski and Gigerenzer, 2012) – to illustrate how a society can change health inequities by changing the activities and policies within each level of the societal infrastructure.

Indeed, a general health policy focuses on the idea of following a healthy diet, taking part in regular exercise, and reducing or eliminating substance use, which includes but is not limited to tobacco, marijuana, and alcohol, to achieve optimal health and reduce morbidity and mortality. Given that it is easy to monitor and measure these behaviors using standardized estimators and comparisons to cohorts made up of similar individuals, in the broader context of health, these behaviors reflect a downstream approach and focus on changing behaviors of the individual, the micro-level approach (Short and Mollborn, 2015). Unfortunately, many of the downstream health-promoting activities are short-lived because of challenges at the meso and macro levels.

In comparison, the social determinants of health that consider changes at the root of social structures which have an influence on societal change, such as policies to ensure equity of income distribution, education, and basic human rights – safety, shelter, and food security – reflect upstream approaches and thereby act at the macro-level (Short and Mollborn, 2015). Upstream approaches are much more difficult to process in society because they are most often dependent on changing the understanding, attitudes, and actions of policymakers, which, in turn, would have a direct impact on changing rules within a society (McMahon, 2022). For the most part, strategies designed to influence the social determinants of health are unbeknownst in terms of target outcomes and generally are reactive to community needs. These strategies may include access to healthcare, provision of employment, and creating a living environment for the unhoused. Such strategies may be described more accurately as "midstream" factors because they are shaped by the jurisdiction in which they can be enacted (Raphael and Brassolotto, 2015). Herein, health-promoting activities reflect reactions that are applied as community programs to the micro level of society by public health servants within local health authorities. When these activities are formulated, directed, and managed by government mandates, they represent activities at the meso and macro levels (Short and Mollborn, 2015; Raphael and Brassolotto, 2015; McMahon, 2022).

Creating a system that is intentional in striving to improve population health in the domains of social, physical, economic, and mental health and which transcends the categories of micro, meso, and macro levels, ensures a more effective and sustainable approach to addressing health inequities and reducing poor health within the population.

As members of society, we have a social responsibility to contribute positively to the health of our community. What this means is that we are responsible for ensuring that the people, the environment, and the conditions to enable a healthy life are achieved by all members of our society. Therefore, to achieve a healthy society, we need to lift every citizen to a suitable threshold across the social determinants of health. Our attention needs to shift so that we focus our efforts on bolstering and sustaining determinants of health rather than simply measuring health outcomes. Population health is conditional on the strides we make with respect to the determinants of health and health inequities.

4.2.1 Income

Links between poverty and health have been observed for centuries. Relations between socioeconomic factors and health often follow a stepwise gradient, with health improving incrementally as social position rises. Such a dose–response relationship may be indicative of a causal role for social factors in determining health outcomes. However, as health scientists, we know that it is difficult to establish causation. In fact, some researchers have suggested reverse causation (Greer et al., 2019; Banack et al., 2019) because of the influence of confounding variables that are interpreted as occurring in reverse order to what may be expected. In the social context of determinants of health, while we may measure the loss of income as leading to poor health outcomes, we can also consider the scenario to be that in which poor health affects the ability to attain a stable income or acquire an adequate education. Yet there is considerable evidence for socioeconomic factors to be recognized as causal agents rather than as merely outcomes. Although health theoretically could limit socioeconomic status, links between education and health cannot be explained by reverse causation because, once attained, educational level is never reduced, and education and income are reliably correlated. Further, research employing longitudinal designs, statistical modeling, and quasi-experiments have all provided evidence for the role of social factors in predicting wide-ranging health outcomes.

Wealth and income, including wages, work-related benefits, and employment status, have a direct influence on an individual's health and also have a direct influence on the inequity among individuals in a society. As noted by Cesarini and colleagues (2016), the health–income gradient is robust and observable among various cohorts. For example, among children from low-income households, there is a greater likelihood that they will be born prematurely and/or weigh less at birth. In addition, children from low-income families are at a higher risk to develop chronic diseases over their lifespan. Conversely, higher household income in childhood is positively associated with better long-term health. The influences of low socioeconomic status extend beyond childhood development. For instance, among older adults, functional impairment occurs along a socioeconomic gradient (Minkler et al., 2006), meaning that those in the lower socioeconomic classes within a given society are more likely to present with issues of functional impairment.

Researchers (Rosenthal et al., 2012; Reine et al., 2013; Norström et al., 2014) indicate that loss of income from unemployment and low income from underemployment are associated with poor health – both physical and mental – and also with lifestyle and behavior choices that are contrary to achieving positive health outcomes. Among unemployed individuals, there is an increase in behavioral risk factors such as overconsumption of substances (alcohol and tobacco), sedentary lifestyle, and increased consumption of low-nutrient foods associated with cardiovascular disease. Moreover, several research studies have reported that unemployment is associated with depression, depressive symptoms, and an increase in perceived life stress related to loss of income from job loss. And while these effects have been observed in the general population, studies have shown that the effects of unemployment and underemployment differ between males and females and that specific sub-cohorts within the population, depending on age, gender, and marital status, are more likely to display negative health consequences of income loss.

Obviously, the most effective way to establish an income is by maintaining stable employment in an environment in which the working conditions are safe and secure. Bringing home an income as a result of maintaining employment not only enhances one's financial decision-making within the marketplace, but it also has a direct impact on an individual's mental and physical health by enhancing self-esteem, lifestyle choices, and societal status and reducing financial stress. In this way, losing the ability to maintain a living wage as a result of unemployment is a precursor to increased morbidity and mortality.

4.3 A Basic Income Guarantee

So what if the government ensured a basic income for all citizens within a community? In 1974, the Canadian federal government and the provincial government of Manitoba created an experiment which came to be known as "Mincome." The formal title was the Manitoba Basic Income Experiment, and it was designed to provide all citizens of Dauphin, Manitoba, a small rural town 300 kilometers northwest of Winnipeg, with a guaranteed annual income when a family's household income fell below the threshold of a low-income cut-off (LICO). The approach was described as a complete saturation experiment in which every family was eligible to receive a designated level of financial support if their employment/income situation was deemed necessary. Follow-up research by Forget (2011, 2013) suggested that, in general, positive outcomes resulted from the establishment of a guaranteed annual income for eligible families. In her retrospective analysis of data from the Mincome experiment, Forget (2013) identified an 8.5% reduction in hospitalizations among study participants from 1974 to 1979. This decline in the need for health services translated to an overall reduction in healthcare costs during the period of observation. While there were several limitations to this political project at the time, as well as the constraints in translating the events of the 1970s Canadian economy to the current situation, the authors support the contention that a guaranteed annual income is good for one's health.

Fast forward to the current day and the fall out of economies devastated by the COVID-19 pandemic. Guaranteed financial support during the pandemic was recognized as a necessary expenditure by governments to maintain free-market economies, such as those in Australia, Canada, and the United States. Direct payments to eligible individuals were necessary to ensure that families maintained access to food and shelter. Yet these programs were temporary and did not have long-term sustainability policies entrenched within the relief strategy. At best, these income supports were short-term measures provided to households that suffered job losses due to the pandemic, and in no way were they demonstrative of planned guaranteed annual income schemes.

> **Implementation of a guaranteed annual income is indeed a wicked problem.**

Research evidence supports that providing a guaranteed annual income can improve self-esteem and reduce the stigma associated with living below the poverty line. However, research by Raphael et al. (2019) suggested that merely providing a basic income guarantee without providing concomitant support for essential social programs would not optimize the potential health advantages that may be anticipated from the introduction of such income support. As a stimulus to lift individuals out of poverty, a guaranteed annual income has merit. Providing financial support for families can reduce the risk of food insecurity and enable a greater potential to access appropriate shelter. However, as noted by Martin and Caminada (2011), there are also negative implications for the implementation of such a social support system. Introducing a guaranteed annual income will have an annual cost burden in the billions of dollars, as exemplified by the financial support provided during the COVID-19 pandemic. Likewise, providing a guaranteed income without restrictions or regulations for eligibility has the potential to reduce the number of individuals in the labor force. Finally, based on reviews of previous experimental guaranteed annual income programs, there is a need to monitor the impacts of such support on family composition, childcare, and distribution of labor within a household.

Clearly, the associations that underlie the availability and distribution of income, employment, and health are complex, as are the results of introducing guaranteed annual income support. The downstream implications of such support have both benefits and consequences that affect our societies and our economies, each of which adds to the complexity of this wicked problem.

4.4 Childhood Development and Early Adversity

As we have seen, low income has detrimental health effects in adulthood, but it also has long-lasting health effects on children raised in poverty. For instance, links between household income in childhood and cognitive function in adulthood have been well established. However, Evans and Schamberg (2009) found that this association is not solely due to the deficits associated with a low-income household but is also explained by exposure to chronic stress. With it, low income brings stress resulting from struggles to sustain food security, housing, childcare, and more. Low income is also a risk factor for mental health and substance use problems among parents, which can shape parenting behaviors and parent–child attachment. In their research, Evans and Schamberg illustrated the effects of the burden of chronic stress, also known as allostatic load, by showing that negative consequences result from the exposure to prolonged chronic stress as a child and the development of working memory as a young adult.

Some of the best-known work on the outcomes of early adversity has been driven by a partnership between the Centers for Disease Control and Kaiser Permanente in research on the enduring consequences of childhood abuse, neglect, and family dysfunction. Referred to as the ACE study aka the Adverse Childhood Experiences Study (Felitti et al., 1998; Gilgoff et al., 2020), this work has proven to be some of the most compelling on the topic of early-life challenges and later-life health. The original ACE study was conducted by surveying adults in two specific sampling distributions (1996 and 1997). In the initial wave of the survey distribution, more than 13,400 adults were recruited to respond to questions about childhood abuse and household dysfunction, as well as to indicate their perceived current health status. The actual participation rate – the number of individuals that completed the first survey and for which their data were included in subsequent analyses – was approximately 59% of eligible individuals. Later reports by Felitti (2002) indicate the original ACE scores were based on a cohort of more than 17,000 adults reporting on experiencing childhood physical abuse, sexual abuse, emotional abuse, parental substance misuse, parental mental illness, domestic violence, and/or imprisonment of a family member. Since the initial study, emotional neglect, physical neglect, and parental divorce were added as categories of adversity, leading to a maximum ACE score of 10. Findings from the original study and subsequent research have connotations for how we deliver healthcare, develop social policies, and define public health.

What the researchers reported was that ACEs are common, that they have a strong and cumulative effect on health and well-being, and that they are major determinants of health. For example, Garrido et al. (2018) reported that individuals with four or more ACES, compared to respondents with none, had a higher likelihood to be involved in violent behavior, engage in substance use, engage in delinquency, and demonstrate any high-risk behavior. Similarly, Rariden et al. (2021) reported that infants born to mothers that reported four or more ACES scores were five times more likely to demonstrate poor emotional and physical health by the time they were only 18 months of age.

ACEs also exert a graded effect on behaviors such as smoking, as Felitti (2002) noted the direct positive correlation between smoking status and ACES scores, meaning that the higher the ACES score the greater the likelihood of smoking. Moreover, these types of relationships also support that the higher the ACES score the greater likelihood of developing ischemic heart disease, cancer, lung disease, and liver disease. Specifically, Felitti (2002) reported that their data showed that a person scoring four or more on

ACES was more likely to develop chronic obstructive pulmonary disease (COPD), and similarly, a person scoring four or more on ACES was as much as 12 times more likely to report depression symptoms and suicidal ideation along with drug and alcohol dependency (Webster, 2022).

Perhaps it should not be surprising that early adversity predicts later disease, given the reported statistical likelihood associated with high ACES scores and involvement in risky health behaviors, such as substance and alcohol use, most likely because these behaviors are strategies used to cope with the allostatic load.[2] However, even when these behavioral risk factors are taken into account, ACEs continue to predict many of the leading causes of morbidity and early mortality (Duffy et al., 2018).

There are measurable physiological reasons why early adversity predicts later-life health. When the body's stress system – or hypothalamic pituitary adrenal (HPA) axis – is chronically activated (Dunlavey, 2018), it has far-reaching effects on other systems, including the nervous system, the immune system, and the endocrine system (Yehuda, 2001; Yaribeygi et al., 2017). Of course, chronic stress affects many biological systems regardless of the life stage in which it is experienced; however, strife and stress in the early years appear to be especially damaging, as they occur in a developing brain and body. When an individual's stress response is persistently activated, we see physiological changes across a number of bodily systems, including the stress system, the immune system, the endocrine system, the nervous system, and the cardiovascular system, in the process known as allostasis. The measurable physiological shift in these systems (the allostatic load) can be quantified in the form of a number of biomarkers, including inflammatory markers, immune cell counts, cardiovascular measures, and indicators of cellular aging (such as DNA methylation and telomere shortening). As such, the allostatic load that accompanies chronic stress may act as a common pathway linking social determinants to disease.

A plethora of studies in several countries have associated adverse childhood experiences and long-term negative health outcomes. However, as indicated by Hertler and coworkers (2022), these associations are not causal but correlated, a clarification with an important implication. Being correlated only indicates that the two measures (overall ACE score and presence of an outcome) are moving in the same direction statistically. It does not mean that reporting adverse childhood experiences guarantees a long-term negative health outcome (Larkin and Cairns, 2020). Despite the fact that there are typically cascading events during the developmental process, there is always the likelihood that the adult will not demonstrate the same behavioral outcome as the parent.

4.5 Race, Racism, and Health Disparities

Race is a social construct (Williams et al., 2019; Macias-Konstantopoulos et al., 2023) and yet race has consistently been associated with health inequities because individuals within a given socially constructed race fall short on the social determinants of health. As noted by Macias-Konstantopoulos and coworkers, Black, Indigenous, and people of color (BIPOC) more often deal with negative issues related to housing and food security. They are also more likely to be exposed to higher-risk environments, and they are more likely to have poor access to healthcare. Similarly, race-related health inequities persist even in countries with universal access to medical care and in programs that strive for equitable healthcare across racial and ethnic groups (Ananth et al., 2001). Williams and colleagues (2019) showed that racism, and specifically structural racism, is a social determinant of health that both adversely and explicitly influences individuals. Moreover, structural racism is persistent, and its effects are measurable within cohorts. Structural racism is the stimulus that leads to different levels of risk as well as inhibited access to opportunities if not resources that enable individuals to achieve positive states of health and well-being.

Race-related lifetime stress exposure (LSE), including racial discrimination and violence and the chronic stress associated with those experiences, the allostatic load, has been identified as an explanatory factor for race-related health inequities that go above and beyond traditional social factors. Race-related stress can lead to negative health outcomes through a variety of mechanisms. For instance, it may lead to unhealthy coping mechanisms, such as using substances as a way of dealing with the trauma of discrimination or race-related violence. In some cases, systemic racism acts as a barrier to higher education, secure employment, and culturally safe healthcare, creating a sense of hopelessness and fatigue around pursuing the means to improve one's social health. Racism may more directly impact health through complex physiological mechanisms whereby chronic activation of the stress system impedes the ability for other physiological systems to function normally.

Considering the dynamics of the COVID-19 crisis, there is ample evidence of specific populations being disproportionately affected. The COVID-19 pandemic compounded many socioeconomic disparities and, in turn, led to more health inequities for people of color. In the U.S., Black and Indigenous communities had the highest per-capita COVID-related hospitalization and death rates. In Canada, the disproportionate influence of COVID-19 was most obvious in Indigenous populations. Although pathogens like COVID-19 do not discriminate, the epidemiology of the disease continues to be shaped by the conditions of the communities affected.

So why are specific populations and communities of color experiencing more dire outcomes? For years, Indigenous communities around the world, faced social and economic injustices that have manifested as health adversities, such as increased prevalence of cardiovascular disease, food insecurity, crowded living arrangements, and lack of clean drinking water, to name but a few examples. Structural racism continues to contribute to inequitable education, employment, and healthcare opportunities among BIPOC. Adverse living conditions and underhousing leave specific populations more susceptible to disease transmission and disease burden. Overcrowding, lack of access to clean water, and shortages of resources for quality daily living within a community, including but not isolating healthcare shortages, constrain one's ability to achieve positive social determinants of health.

Social determinants affect health and contribute to health inequities, and without question, racism is a precursor to health disparities. While the social determinants of health provide a good starting point to consider the influences of social constructs on the health of communities and their individuals, there is a need to continue exploring the complexities of the determinants. As Frank and coworkers (2020) suggested, there is a need to rethink the social determinants of health in light of the *complexity and wickedness of public health problems*. What remains less clear is by what mechanism social, political, and economic factors promote or deter the attainment of positive determinants of health.

Can a discussion of the social determinants of health occur without investigating the importance of resilience of the individual, the community, or the population?

The notion that social determinants lead to disease through biological mechanisms indicates a need to integrate social and biological perspectives of health while also considering the importance of resilience. Whereas social lenses alone may struggle to explain why individuals from very similar life circumstances show divergent health outcomes, biomedical lenses reveal how the same stressors can trigger different neurophysiological responses across individuals. For example, biological response to the same stressor can vary markedly depending on the presence or absence of specific genetic conditions. As we have seen, relationships between social factors and health are complex and interactive; they may involve mechanisms implicating various biological systems, and at times, they may only manifest decades after exposure to the social determinant.

4.6 Conclusion

What is the value of understanding the social determinants of health?

The role of social factors in health is undeniable, and this role needs to be investigated, yet not merely to quantify the number of factors that influence health or to qualify whether the determinant has been achieved positively. Rather, we must do so to determine the complexity of the determinant – that is, to understand all of the nuances of social determinants as they influence health and well-being (Rose et al., 2008). Only then can a truly integrative and comprehensive approach to improving the health of a population be achieved.

4.6.1 Discussion Questions

1 Define the term *salutogenesis*. How does salutogenesis relate to the concept of well-being? What are the social determinants of health that fit best with the concept of salutogenesis?

2 The social determinants of health were presented in this chapter as a list of considerations, but the order was not ranked. How would you rank the items presented in the list? Provide your rationale.

3 ACES are real. However, the early work on ACES was completed in the United States and with very specific cohorts of individuals and families. How might the early work to develop the concept of ACES influence the knowledge translation of ACES to a different country?

Notes

1 A latent variable is a variable that is not measured directly but results from a mathematical approach that produces the estimator by combining measures in an analytical process. Latent variables can be generated through such procedures as factor analysis, principal component analysis, and structural equation modeling.

2 *Allostatic load* is the term used to describe the effects of chronic stress on an individual that leads to a measurable negative physiological outcome (Rodriquez et al., 2019).

References

Ananth CV, Misra DP, Demissie K, Smulian JC. Rates of preterm delivery among Black women and White women in the United States over two decades: An age-period-cohort analysis. *Am J Epidemiol*. 2001;154(7):657–665.

Banack HR, Bea JW, Kaufman JS, et al. The effects of reverse causality and selective attrition on the relationship between body mass index and mortality in postmenopausal women. *Am J Epidemiol*. 2019;188(10):1838–1848. doi:10.1093/aje/kwz160

Bautista TG, Roman G, Khan M, et al. What is well-being? A scoping review of the conceptual and operational definitions of occupational well-being. *J Clin Transl Sci*. 2023;7:e227. doi:10.1017/cts.2023.648.

Bell N, Wilkerson R, Mayfield-Smith K, Lòpez-De Fede A. Community social determinants and health outcomes drive availability of patient-centered medical homes. *Health Place*. 2021;67:102439. doi:10.1016/j.healthplace.2020.102439

Cesarini D, Lindqvist E, Östling R, Wallace B. Wealth, health, and child development: Evidence from administrative data on Swedish lottery players. *Quart J Econ*. 2016;131(2):687–738.

Duffy KA, McLaughlin KA, Green PA. Early life adversity and health-risk behaviors: Proposed psychological and neural mechanisms. *Ann N Y Acad Sci*. 2018;1428(1):151–169. doi:10.1111/nyas.13928

Dunlavey CJ. Introduction to the hypothalamic-pituitary-adrenal axis: Healthy and dysregulated stress responses, developmental stress and neurodegeneration. *J Undergrad Neurosci Educ*. 2018;16(2):R59–R60.

Evans GW, Schamberg MA. Childhood poverty, chronic stress, and adult working memory. *Proc Nat Acad Sci*. 2009;106(16), 6545–6549. doi:10.1073/pnas.0811910106

Felitti VJ. The relation between adverse childhood experiences and adult health: Turning gold into lead. *Perm J*. 2002;6(1):44–47. doi:10.7812/TPP/02.994

Felitti VJ, Anda RF, Nordenberg D, et al. Relationship of childhood abuse and household dysfunction to many of the leading causes of death in adults. The Adverse Childhood Experiences (ACE) Study. *Am J Prev Med*. 1998;14(4):245–258. doi:10.1016/s0749-3797(98)00017-8

Forget EL. The town with no poverty: The health effects of a Canadian guaranteed annual income field experiment. *Canadian Public Policy*. 2011;37:283–305.

Forget EL. New questions, new data, old interventions: The health effects of a guaranteed annual income. *Prev Med*. 2013;57(6):925–928.

Frank J, Abel T, Campostrini S, Cook S, Lin VK, McQueen DV. The social determinants of health: Time to re-think? *Int J Environ Res Pub Health*. 2020;17(16). doi:10.3390/ijerp7165856

Garrido EF, Weiler LM, Taussig HN. Adverse childhood experiences and health-risk behaviors in vulnerable early adolescents. *J Early Adolesc*. 2018;38(5):661–680. doi:10.1177/0272431616687671

Gilgoff R, Singh L, Koita K, Gentile B, Marques SS. Adverse childhood experiences, outcomes, and interventions. *Pediatr Clin North Am*. 2020;67(2):259–273. doi:10.1016/j.pcl.2019.12.001

Graham H. Social determinants and their unequal distribution: Clarifying policy understandings. *Mil Quart*. 2004;82(1):101–124.

Greer FR, Sicherer SH, Burks AW. The effects of early nutritional interventions on the development of atopic disease in infants and children: The role of maternal dietary restriction, breastfeeding, hydrolyzed formulas, and timing of introduction of allergenic complementary foods. *Pediatrics*. 2019;143(4):e20190281. doi:10.1542/peds.2019-0281

Hertler S, de Baca TC, Peñaherrera-Aguirre M, et al. Life history evolution forms the foundation of the *Adverse Childhood Experience* pyramid. *Evol Psychol Sci* 2022;8:89–104. doi:10.1007/s40806-021-00299-5

Islam MM. Social determinants of health and related inequalities: Confusion and Implications. *Front Pub Health*. 2019;7:11.

Jarden A, Roache A. What is well-being? *Int J Environ Res Public Health*. 2023;20(6):5006. doi:10.3390/ijerph20065006

Larkin W, Cairns P. Addressing adverse childhood experiences: Implications for professional practice. *Br J Gen Pract*. 2020;70(693):160–161.

Macias-Konstantopoulos WL, Collins KA, Diaz R, et al. Race, healthcare, and health disparities: A critical review and recommendations for advancing health equity. *West J Emerg Med.* 2023;24(5):906–918. doi:10.5811/westjem.58408

Marewski JN, Gigerenzer G. Heuristic decision making in medicine. *Dialogues Clin Neurosci.* 2012;14(1):77–89. doi:10.31887/DCNS.2012.14.1/jmarewski

Martin MC, Caminada K. Welfare reform in the US: A policy overview analysis. *Poverty Pub Pol.* 2011;3(1):1–38.

McMahon NE. Framing action to reduce health inequalities: What is argued for through use of the 'upstream – downstream' metaphor? *J Pub Health.* 2022;44(3):671–678. doi:10.1093/pubmed/fdab157

Minkler M, Fuller-Thomson E, Guralnik JM. Gradient of disability across the socioeconomic spectrum in the United States. *N Engl J Med.* 2006;355(7):695–703.

Mittelmark MB. Introduction to the handbook of salutogenesis. In: Mittelmark MB, Sagy S, Eriksson M, et al., editors. *The Handbook of Salutogenesis.* Cham: Springer; 2017. doi:10.1007/978-3-319-04600-6_1

Mittelmark MB, Bauer GF, Vaandrager L, et al., editors. Salutogenesis as a theory, as an orientation and as the sense of coherence. In *The Handbook of Salutogenesis.* Cham: Springer; 2022.

Norström F, Virtanen P, Hammarström A, Gustafsson PE, Janlert U. How does unemployment affect self-assessed health? A systematic review focusing on subgroup effects. *BMC Pub Health.* 2014;14(1):1–13.

Raphael D, Brassolotto J. Understanding action on the social determinants of health: A critical realist analysis of in-depth interviews with staff of nine Ontario public health units. *BMC Res Notes.* 2015;8:105. doi:10.1186/s13104-015-1064-5

Raphael D, Bryant T, Mendly-Zambo Z. Canada considers a basic income guarantee: Can it achieve health for all? *Health Promot Int.* 2019;34(5):1025–1031.

Rariden C, SmithBattle L, Yoo JH, Cibulka N, Loman D. Screening for adverse childhood experiences: Literature review and practice implications. *J Nurse Pract.* 2021;17(1):98–104. doi:10.1016/j.nurpra.2020.08.002

Reine I, Novo M, Hammarström A. Unemployment and ill health – a gender analysis: Results from a 14-year follow-up of the Northern Swedish Cohort. *Pub Health.* 2013;127(3):214–222.

Rhodes T, Singer M, Bourgois P, Friedman SR, Strathdee SA. The social structural production of HIV risk among injecting drug users. *Soc Sci Med.* 2005;61(5):1026–1044. doi:10.1016/j.Socscimed.2004.12.024

Rodriquez EJ, Kim EN, Sumner AE, Nápoles AM, Pérez-Stable EJ. Allostatic load: Importance, markers, and score determination in minority and disparity populations. *J Urban Health.* 2019;96(Suppl 1):3–11. doi:10.1007/s11524-019-00345-5

Rose G, Khaw K, Marmot M. *Rose's Strategy of Preventive Medicine.* Oxford: Oxford University Press; 2008.

Rosenthal L, Carroll-Scott A, Earnshaw VA, Santilli A, Ickovics JR. The importance of full-time work for urban adults' mental and physical health. *Soc Sci Med.* 2012;75(9):1692–1696.

Short SE, Mollborn S. Social determinants and health behaviors: Conceptual frames and empirical advances. *Curr Opin Psychol.* 2015;5:78–84. doi:10.1016/j.copsyc.2015.05.002

Simons G, Baldwin DS. A critical review of the definition of 'well-being' for doctors and their patients in a post Covid-19 era. *Int J Soc Psychiat.* 2021;67(8):984–991.

Thimm-Kaiser M, Benzekri A, Guilamo-Ramos V. Conceptualizing the mechanisms of social determinants of health: A heuristic framework to inform future directions for mitigation. *Mil Quart.* 2023;101:486–526. doi:10.1111/1468-0009.12642

US Department of Health and Human Services Healthy People 2030 Agenda. Office of Disease Prevention and Health Promotion. Available at: https://health.gov/healthypeople/objectives-and-data/social-determinants-health/literature-summaries/health-literacy

Webster EM. The impact of adverse childhood experiences on health and development in young children. *Glob Pediatr Health.* 2022;9. doi:10.1177/2333794X221078708

Williams DR, Lawrence JA, Davis BA. Racism and health: Evidence and needed research. *Annu Rev Public Health*. 2019;40:105–125. doi:10.1146/annurev-publhealth-040218-043750

World Health Organization. *Closing the Gap in a Generation: Health Equity through Action on the Social Determinants of Health*. Final Report of the Commission on Social Determinants of Health; 2008.

World Health Organization. *Health Promotion Glossary of Terms 2021*. Geneva: World Health Organization; 2021. License: CC BY-NC-SA 3.0IGO. Retrieved from 9789240038349-eng.pdf (who.int) on January 2024.

Yaribeygi H, Panahi Y, Sahraei H, Johnston TP, Sahebkar A. The impact of stress on body function: A review. *Excli J*. 2017;16:1057–1072. doi:10.17179/excli2017-480

Yehuda R. Biology of post traumatic stress disorder. *J Clin Psychiat*. 2001;62(suppl 17):41–46.

CHAPTER 5

On the Importance of Health Literacy

5.0 Introduction

When we consider literacy, we are not thinking merely in a sense about whether an individual can read or write. Rather, we are referring to an individual's ability to read, to write, to work with numerals, and to understand information and to process information in a functional way. Understanding is a central tenet in the development of knowledge. We can, therefore, refer to literacy as the level of proficiency at which an individual can use information to function in society.

Yet how we define the term literacy is important to constructing statistics that represent the population of literate individuals. For example, in 2020, the report to the United Nations General Assembly[1] the United Nations Educational, Scientific and Cultural Organization (UNESCO) stated that the "the global adult literacy rate for the population aged 15 years and older was 86 per cent in 2018." Yet the report also indicated that the number of illiterate individuals grew from some 23 million to more than 773 million people. Moreover, these figures do not simply reflect who can read, write, or work with numerals but also whether these individuals have continued to develop these skills in a constantly expanding global marketplace that requires contextual application of these skills to advance. As noted in the report, with increased digitization and globalization, individuals will need to develop new literacies, as in working with the new forms of communication and the ubiquity of artificial intelligence across all realms of society. Advances in industry and new methods of production of goods and services will require continued personal growth and development of new skills that require such new literacies. Likewise, given the increasing flow of migrants across borders and into areas that once held a lingua franca that was regionally sacrosanct, we can now add the need to develop multilingualism to the skill set of expanding literacies. Finally, we need to think of literacy on a continuum, where the basic skills of reading, writing, and numeracy are simply a starting point. The disparities across social classes, be they implicit or explicit, are directly reflective of the spectrum of literacy within any region on the planet.

DOI: 10.4324/9781003474777-5

For example, despite all our good feelings about Canada, nearly half[2] of the population of Canadians between the ages of 16 and 65 is considered to have low literacy skills. As noted in *the Programme for the International Assessment of Adult Competencies* (PIAAC, 2013), Canada has a mixed rating on the indicators that are used to assess a nation's level of literacy, numeracy, and the ability to solve problems in a technology-rich environment. PIAAC is a survey conducted by the Organisation for Economic Cooperation and Development (OECD), and it is intended to measure among adults their proficiency in information processing that includes literacy, numeracy and information processing, and, more importantly, how the respondents use these skills in various settings that include their home, their workplace, and the external community.[3] The PIAAC report indicated that in comparison to other countries in the OECD, Canada scored only average on our levels of literacy, below average on our proficiency in numeracy, but above average in our abilities to solve problems in a technology-rich environment – the latter category is referred to as PS-TRE (problem-solving in technology-rich environments).

Yet this is not surprising, because for many Canadians, their normal work life does not require them to be challenged with tasks that require critical thinking, reading for deeper understanding, or writing to express themselves. For a portion of Canadians, their daily lives may not require any interaction with literacy skills, resulting in a lack of motivation to change their literacy proficiency. These data are important in that the survey results not only compare Canada to the other 24 countries from the OECD that participated in the survey in 2012 but also demonstrate the differences in these scores across provinces within Canada and, most notably, across selected cohorts that comprise the population. That is, according to the results of the first PIAAC report, minority cohorts, which were comprised of immigrants and Indigenous persons, had high variability in the scores on each of literacy, numeracy, and PS-TRE and, as such, warranted further research on possible causal mechanisms for such outcomes.

Although the UNESCO estimate for the world to have achieved 86% adult literacy may seem like a major accomplishment, it does not reflect the levels of illiteracy among youth, nor does it reflect the distribution of literacy around the globe (Murray, 2021). While it may seem overly cliché to state that children represent the future of our civilization, it is imperative that illiteracy, defined as the inability to read, write, work with numerals, and understand and problem-solve in a highly technological world, be addressed as a critical investment of time and resources. Murray (2021) pointed out that the disruption of the COVID-19 global pandemic has serendipitously enabled us to reconsider how we view the advancement of literacy beyond the written word. According to Murray, educators have an opportunity to rethink the ways in which they engage children to develop skills that can enhance their development of literacy. That is, educators can reset their attention and approaches beyond the traditional teaching proficiency in reading as the "sage on the stage" to incorporating activities that draw on the child's creativity, sharing experiences, including actions that draw on all their senses and integrate technology, not as a substitute for human interaction but as the "guide on the side."

As societies continue to build economies on technology and complex systems of daily engagement, there will be a need for individuals to maintain and, in many cases, enhance their numeracy and literacy skills while improving their understanding of new technologies (Nikou et al., 2022). For example, consider how often during the pandemic your purchases were based on internet searches and your method of payment was digital. Consider also how many more manual labor opportunities were lost in the marketplace in comparison to workforces that were based on digital information processing. Long before the first turn of Johannes Gutenberg's printing press in the 1400s, one could surmise that technology was ubiquitous in human civilization, as was the need to adapt to ever-emerging and ever-evolving technologies. Yet as humans, we are not quick to accept or adjust to changes that require effort of will, stamina, or thinking (Davis, 1989). However, technological changes do not wait for us or for our societies to adjust attitudes and accept change. The ever-evolving landscape of technological change has created new literacies – information literacy, digitization literacy, and media literacy as examples. Here we understand the definition of information literacy to be a developed skill that demonstrates a capability to identify, understand, and utilize information in various processes and presentations (Černý, 2022). Digitization literacy, as noted by Tinmaz et al. (2022), lacks a simple definition but again can be described as a capacity of an individual to not only make sense of information but also to create, evaluate, and use digital information and the effective use of the technology that facilitates the use of digital information (Nikou et al., 2022). Additionally, media literacy, which seems to be the simplest of the literacy types to recognize because of its omnipresence, is also described as an ability to access, analyze, and report information (Schwarz, 2005). Add to these ever-evolving literacies the integration of artificial intelligence literacy as a method by which we can optimize technological advancement, and we see very quickly how the calculus of literacy will show our shortcomings as a society (Selenko et al., 2022).

Artificial intelligence literacy was defined by Long and Magerko (2020) as a set of competencies that consider how individuals view artificial intelligence, especially with regard to public misconceptions, and how individuals can make sense of artificial intelligence. Just as in considering other forms of literacy, artificial intelligence literacy is about people's understanding of artificial intelligence and all its ramifications, given their background, culture, attitude, and lived experiences. Recognizing the potential weaknesses that could arise from artificial intelligence illiteracy among the American population, the U.S. House of Representatives introduced an amendment to the Digital Equity Act of 2021. The bipartisan Artificial Intelligence Literacy Act of 2023[4] was specifically intended to enhance the development of artificial intelligence literacy among the U.S. citizenry as a means to ensure American society could be competitive with other countries in regard to the applications of technology for education, commerce, industry, and, of course, national security.

To suggest that developing literacy is essential would be an understatement, especially given the measurable benefits of basic reading, writing, and numeracy, the value of understanding the information to which we are exposed constantly, and the ability to put into action the knowledge that we derive from the implicit learning that results from being literate. Yet not all individuals are on the shiny road to lifelong wisdom, as noted by the U.K. National Literary Trust,[5] which indicated that in England, 1 in 6 adults or 7.1 million persons were considered to have low basic literacy skills. Likewise, in Scotland, the rate was 1 in 4 or 931,000 people; in Wales, it was 1 in 8 or 216,000 people; and in Northern Ireland, it was 1 in 5 or 256,000 people. While this may seem like only a few individuals given the ever-burgeoning population of the world, these figures reflect a real cost estimate of nearly 55 billion pounds per year to the wider economy of the United Kingdom.[6]

5.1 Defining Health Literacy

The mentioned indicators of adult competencies (i.e., print literacy, numeracy, digital problem-solving) are important antecedents to health literacy (Speros, 2005). After all, being able to read and understand print is important for reviewing and appraising pertinent health information, including product labels, prescriptions, and health pamphlets. Numeracy skills are useful in terms of adhering to the specific dosage of medications or the ability to monitor various health outcomes, such as concentrations of blood glucose or the systolic and diastolic measurements of blood pressure. Similarly, digital literacy can be considered a critical aptitude when requiring a level of understanding to identify reputable sources of health information either from local health authorities within one's community or through an open search on the internet. Having an ability to know what to look for when considering one's health status, whom to ask for support or advice on matters related to health outcomes, and when to steer away from untrustworthy services or information resources are also part of a level of necessary health literacy. But health literacy entails much more than the basic aspects of general literacy. Although there is no consensus regarding a precise definition of health literacy (Liu et al., 2020), most often, definitions of health literacy emphasize an individual's ability to obtain, understand, appraise, and apply information that is specific to maintaining or enhancing one's health (Olisarova et al., 2021). Previous research suggests a lack of health literacy has several negative implications for an individual's overall health outcomes (Coughlin et al., 2020; Liu et al., 2020). Health illiteracy may begin with an inability to comprehend essential information necessary to achieve a positive level of overall health. That is, a lack of comprehension attributed to health illiteracy is a precursor to inappropriate decision-making related to positive health practices like adherence to medication regimens or attending appointments for healthcare, ignoring messaging about lifestyle decisions such as smoking, substance use, exercise, or exposure to adverse environments, along with the greater likelihood of participating in high-risk behaviors (Hickey et al., 2018). While low levels of health literacy can be identified among cohorts of individuals across all levels of society (Prince et al., 2018), in the United States, low health literacy was most likely to be associated with individuals who were older, individuals that had a low level of education, and individuals that were in the lower income strata. Likewise, low levels of health literacy have also been identified among individuals classified as having a chronic condition as well as those individuals whose first language is not English (Hickey et al., 2018; Coughlin et al., 2020; Liu et al., 2020; Stormacq et al., 2020).

Based on a thorough systematic review and qualitative synthesis of related research literature on the topic of health literacy, Liu and colleagues (2020) suggested that health literacy can be summarized by three important features. First is the capacity to develop appropriate knowledge of the systems that deliver health services. Second is the ability to process essential information in relation to health constructs and the provision of healthcare. Third is an understanding of the importance of both self-management and working with health providers to maintain one's health. Each of these themes has been well supported in the literature, and despite different research objectives, the messages across studies are similar. For example, with respect to knowledge, researchers describe this trait as demonstrating an understanding of the healthcare system and an individual's ability to identify the important information that has direct implications for their health. Moreover, as noted by Protheroe et al. (2009), individuals with higher levels of health literacy are more likely to be directly involved in healthcare decisions about their well-being and longer-term outcomes.

Having an ability to process essential information in relation to specific health constructs and especially those directly related to the provision of healthcare that an individual could receive was exemplified by the tragic scenario presented by Nielsen-Bohlman et al. (2004). Here, the authors described the outcome for a patient that visited a hospital with fever and abdominal pain, and she was told that she was being scheduled for an exploratory laparotomy. Not fully understanding what the procedure was or what it could do for her, she left the hospital angry and told the staff that she was in pain and all they wanted to do was an exploratory. In actuality, an exploratory laparotomy is a surgical procedure that opens up the abdomen to identify the cause of pain or bleeding which could not be otherwise diagnosed.[7] Unfortunately, the patient later died after returning home with appendicitis.

Realizing that we are responsible for our health outcomes is a product of achieving higher health literacy. Being able to self-manage our conditions with the support of healthcare providers is necessary in optimizing our potential well-being. Paterick and coworkers (2017) describe the value of promoting self-management of one's health, enhancing patient education, and establishing partnerships between healthcare providers and their partners. For example, based on an estimate of risk known as a hazard ratio – which compares groups relative to change or survival outcomes – Ford et al. (2009) found that when individuals didn't smoke, maintained a low body mass index, ate healthfully, and participated in regular exercise, they were as much as 78% less likely to develop diabetes, myocardial infarction, stroke, or cancer, compared to cohorts that smoked, ate foods that were contrary to healthy food guides, did not maintain a healthy mass, and lived sedentary lives.

In simplest terms, individuals need to maintain a level of health literacy that will ensure that they can "obtain, process, and understand information" for appropriate decisions related to their health (Zegers et al., 2020). In fact, according to Güner and Ekmekci (2019), in comparison to other social determinants of health, such as ethnicity, employment, income, and education levels, the authors believe that health literacy is the strongest predictor of an individual's health status. Although we cannot discount the impact of externalities such as early life experiences and economic, social, and environmental factors, there remains a unique pathway between health literacy and health-impacting behaviors, such as smoking, sedentary living, and the recreational use of alcohol and other substances. Hence the need for continued health education and health-promoting programs that help to mitigate the negative health consequences of low health literacy.

Research in the province of British Columbia by Kwan and coworkers (2006) suggested that health literacy is influenced by the social determinants of health in that it is directly linked to health education, and later research by DeMarco and Nystrom (2010) also supported the contention that health literacy was directly related to health education. Consequently, health literacy can also be considered in and of itself as a determinant of health because of its influence as a motivator to seek support, its importance to understanding health status consequences, and its influence on personal decision-making with regard to specific actions that can lead to measurable health outcomes.

Improving health communication may have critical implications for increasing health literacy. However, as we recognize the uniqueness of societies, we are learning more about the humiliation that social and political structures have forced on even simple events like seeking healthcare. For example, overcoming the stigma associated with not knowing information that some feel should be common knowledge and the related feelings of failure from this lack of knowledge is an important consideration in understanding the relationship between health communication and health literacy. Aldoory (2017) described the use of health communication not only to inform the public but also to empower the public from two distinct perspectives. The first approach is a combination of "targeting and tailoring" in which specific health messages are designed for specific groups of individuals (targeted) to ensure that they can be read, understood, and acted on by cohorts with perceived levels of health literacy. In this approach, the messages are structured, presented, and communicated so as to ensure that they appeal to the characteristics of the targeted sample (tailored). The second approach that Aldoory described was called the "universal precautions approach." In this approach, there is an implicit assumption that the population has a low level of literacy, and it is therefore the responsibility of the information provider to ensure that the message is "clear, culturally sensitive, and appropriate" for the intended cohort (DeMarco and Nystrom, 2010).

A compromise to these two paradigms of health communication is through what is referred to as communicative health literacy. The communicative health literacy approach recognizes the complexity inherent in developing health literacy across different cohorts. As Aldoory (2017) explained, through a communicative health literacy approach, the construct of health literacy is "co-constructed" between the individual and the health information broker in such a way as to respect the social background of the individual. By respecting the position of the individual as an information recipient, an implicit collaboration between the source of information and the recipient of information will establish an interaction that represents a shared understanding of the health literacy level within the communication. By establishing this interactional relationship, Aldoory stated that the information broker has given agency to the information recipient and thereby increased the likelihood for the individual to act on the information.

Some scholars also believe that a distinction should be made in discussing medical or individual health literacy versus societal or public health literacy (Coughlin et al., 2020). Individually, health literacy attends to the individual's core qualities that shape health-related decision-making and associated clinical outcomes, such as longevity, health services use, and motivation to engage in pro-health behaviors. Public health literacy, on the other hand, involves the same conceptual dimensions as medical health literacy but applies to a larger group or community. As such, the outcomes play out on a wider scale and may result in more sophisticated public dialogue around health issues, community empowerment to address social determinants of health, and health inequities, along with social pressure to update public policy in more favorable ways. Viewed from this perspective, improving health literacy levels in society is essential to improving the health of a society.

One of the timeliest examples of health literacy, with applications for disease prevention on a public health scale, is, of course, the public's ability to acquire, understand, and use information related to the spread of disease. Throughout the COVID-19 pandemic, misinformation presented at certain levels of government, especially in the United States (Simoes and Jackson-Thompson, 2023) and Brazil (Ferigato et al., 2020), led to mass confusion and misunderstanding of health outcomes associated with behaviors that not only increased the risk of disease transmission but which also the actual prevalence of cases, hospitalizations, and deaths. Especially in the early days of the pandemic, a lack of understanding about the mechanism of transmission of the virus meant that individuals were unaware of the importance of social distancing, wearing a mask, and self-isolation for presumptive and confirmed cases. The fact that there continues to be a discussion among healthy individuals about whether to accept the vaccine speaks to the lack of understanding about the benefits of widespread immunization on reducing spread, controlling outcomes, and containing viruses.

5.2 On the Importance of Vaccines and Vaccinating the Population to Control Disease Spread

Health literacy about vaccines is essential to ensuring that health authorities can not only flatten the curve – that is, to lower the incidence rate (i.e., the number of new cases within a given time period) so that the number of new cases is spread out over a longer period – but can, in some cases, eliminate the virus from society. Vaccines are not conventional drugs but are "biologics," otherwise known as biologic drugs, which, according to Health Canada, refer to drugs that are derived from living organisms[8] or the cells of living organisms. Biologics are defined as formulations that include an active ingredient, which is either a synthetic form, a dead form, or a weakened form of the disease-causing agent.

This active agent is referred to as the antigen because it contains the material that looks like the disease. Yet because the vaccine is an inert (non-reacting) molecule, it does not begin the harmful destructive mission of self-propagation. Rather, the presence of the vaccine provokes the immune system (the body's defense mechanisms) to produce a type of white blood cell known as a B lymphocyte (LeBien and Tedder, 2008), which, in turn, produces protein molecules called antibodies. Antibodies circulate in the blood, searching for the corresponding antigen. Once the antibody identifies a disease-specific antigen, it will connect to the antigen at a specific receptor site and neutralize or render the antigen non-functional. There are two types of B lymphocyte cells: (i) the plasma cells and (ii) the memory cells (Cano and Lopera, 2013). We can think of the plasma cells as the fast-acting cells that act immediately on the presence of antigens (the bad stuff in our blood) and the memory cells as the detecting cells that continue to search and act on the presence of antigens once we have recovered from the presence of a disease. As such, through inoculation with a vaccine, we establish disease-specific immunity.

Viruses and bacteria are made up of protein structures with distinct shapes. The severe acute respiratory syndrome coronavirus 2 (SARS-CoV-2), which most of the world knows as COVID-19, has at least three specific protein structures on the outer tunic (layer) of the virus that give the molecule a corona or crown-like appearance. Figure 5.1 presents the very recognizable image of the COVID-19 virus. This image shows the protein structures on the outer layer of the COVID-19 molecule.

Vaccines are essential in protecting us from harmful diseases because they assist our immune system by priming it to recognize and eliminate harmful pathogens, such as bacteria or viruses, and differentiate which of the 100 trillion life-forms (bacteria and viruses) – in and on our bodies – are good for us and which can cause illness and even death. Vaccines are essential to maintaining positive states of health because they aid

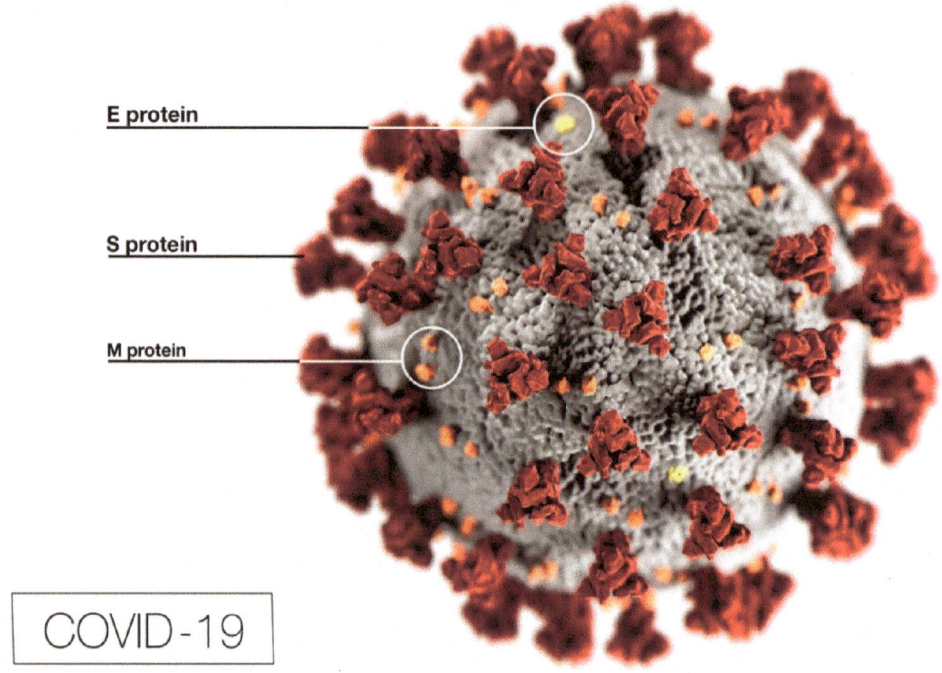

E protein

S protein

M protein

COVID-19

Figure 5.1 CDC image of COVID-19 illustrating the protein tunic of the virus.

our immune system to identify and differentiate the creatures that are good for us from the ones that are intent on perpetuating their own existence without regard for our life. Vaccines can therefore be considered training substances in that they train the immune system to recognize very specific structures of viruses like a coronavirus (COVID-19) and bacteria like the tuberculosis-causing bacteria, *Mycobacterium tuberculosis*.

Prior to COVID-19, the typical vaccine approach was to stimulate the immune system by having a vaccine mimic a pathogen of interest. That is, by presenting a pseudo-pathogen to the blood in the form of a vaccine, the immune system in turn was signaled to begin producing antibodies to search the blood for an antigen. However, during the spread of the COVID-19 pandemic, researchers introduced a new immune system signaling strategy using messenger RNA (mRNA). The molecule mRNA is an intermediary molecule, located between the DNA in the cell nucleus and protein structures residing in the cytoplasm. In a normal process of protein synthesis, the DNA molecule would be uncoiled by specific enzymes, and the coded information of the DNA would be transcribed onto the mRNA molecule within the nucleus of a cell. The mRNA then fulfills its messenger function by exiting the nucleus and translating the DNA code into a protein structure, which it helps to build in the cytoplasm. This process of creating new proteins in the cytoplasm is referred to as protein synthesis.

The role of mRNA as a virus buster is to produce specific proteins of the virus of interest that, in turn, invoke the body's immune response, building a supply of disease-specific antibodies. In COVID-19, the protein of interest is the spike protein. Therefore, the mRNA produces an inactive form of the spike protein that cannot harm the host – that's us! Rather, because the protein produced by the mRNA replicates the spike protein of the virus, we can train the antibodies to attach directly to the spike and thereby knock out the virus's active state. In this way, we can teach the body to control the infection by capitalizing on the virus's own mechanism of propagation.

5.3 Vaccinating Large Samples in the Population and Establishing Herd Immunity Through Health Literacy

Life before the development of vaccines meant that children and young adults were at constant risk of death and infirmity from diseases such as measles, polio, tuberculosis, diphtheria, and rubella. Today, these diseases are considered vaccine preventable and, in developed countries, are virtually non-existent when the population participates in public health immunization programs. The efficacy of immunization requires acceptance and adherence to the recommended behaviors by all eligible individuals in the community. Part of these behaviors include a willingness to practice the public health measures that prevent spread as well as to be immunized against the pathogen by participating in regular vaccination programs. While these resolutions to health maintenance and disease prevention sound simple, they may require a level of health literacy that supports one's understanding of potential positive outcomes for their own health and the health within a community. Often, individuals lack an awareness of these suggested measures or of the rationale behind these suggestions and thus do not participate in the recommended public health processes.

For example, in 1995, Canada adopted a two-dose model of immunization to reduce and eradicate measles in individuals under the age of 17. However, despite the best efforts of public health departments to immunize all those at risk, a super-spreader event occurred in 2011 when there was an importation of the virus from Europe, which, at the time, had more than 30,000 active cases of the virus. The event, which occurred in the province of Quebec, led to a spread of some 725 cases, of which 678 were attributed to a mass transmission through sustained contact between individuals in a community – aka a super-spreader event. When a community accepts the regimen to be inoculated against measles, most physicians will never see a case, but when communities resist such immunization programs, measles outbreaks occur quickly and spread to those who are not protected.

> **When we are immunized, we reduce the risk of pathogen (virus, bacteria) spread, protect those who are vulnerable, and, in many cases, increase the opportunity to eradicate the disease.**

Measles can kill. Why put your child at this unnecessary risk?

In the case of the Quebec outbreak in 2011, the rapid transmission especially among children in the 12-to-17-year age sub-cohort may have been a combination of failure to vaccinate, which reflects the attitudes and behaviors of the population, combined with vaccination failure, which reflects the inability of the vaccine to build appropriate immunity to the virus. However, by improving the rate of immunization using such strategies as two-dose methodologies, we can decrease the risk of disease spread.

The term *herd immunity* refers to the establishment of immunity among a large sample of individuals within a community. By vaccinating communities of individuals, we reduce the risk of becoming infected with the disease and spreading the disease to others. Simply put, through large-scale immunization programs, that is by vaccinating most people in a community, we can establish herd immunity and thereby reduce the spread of the pathogen or disease among individuals within the community. In many communities, there will be a sub-group of individuals that cannot be inoculated because they are too young, have a compromised immune system, or are currently being treated for a specific disease. These individuals need the rest of us to be vaccinated to establish intrinsic protection from the vaccine. Establishing this form of herd immunity depends not only on scientific and clinical readiness (i.e., having adequate supply of a rigorously tested vaccine) but also on public readiness (i.e., intent among a large proportion of the population to be vaccinated). Global health movements have called for the equitable distribution of a COVID-19 vaccine. Part of equitable vaccine distribution is strategic communication to increase confidence among segments of the population who remain vaccine hesitant. When sufficient proportions of the population are immunized, we reduce the risk of transmitting pathogens – viruses and bacteria – and, in many situations, we increase the opportunity to eradicate the disease.

5.4 The Need for Continued Vigilance

Except for smallpox, it is safe to expect that diseases do not die off. In many countries, widespread immunization programs are not possible for a variety of factors, some related to geographical limitations and some because of social determinants, such as widescale poverty. Yet whenever public health programs have instituted community immunization programs, there has been a concomitant decrease in the incidence rate (number of new cases within a defined period) that can lead to significant declines in illness, hospitalizations, life-long infirmity (such as paralysis from polio), and death (De Serres et al., 2013). For example, as noted by Gangarosa et al. (1998):

> Pertussis incidence was 10 to 100 times lower in countries where high vaccine coverage was maintained than in countries where immunization programs were compromised by anti-vaccine movements. Comparisons of neighboring countries with high and low vaccine coverage further underscore the efficacy of these vaccines. Given the safety and cost-effectiveness of whole-cell pertussis vaccines, our study shows that, far from being obsolete, these vaccines continue to have an important role in global immunization. (p. 356)

> **By improving health literacy through specific program promotion and, more specifically, health education, we promote positive change regarding vaccine intentions and vaccine uptake.**
>
> **(Vikram et al., 2012)**

As noted by Abdel-Latif (2020), one of the greatest confounders to a population's understanding of the urgency to act positively toward the control and eradication of the novel coronavirus has been the level of the population's health literacy or the lack thereof. We are now, more than ever, aware of the importance of infectious disease as a major cause of death and disruption in societies. Yet the pandemic has done more than merely expose the risk of death due to infection. The pandemic has exposed the problems related to the health of and the health within our society. As noted by Tai et al. (2021), African American, Native American, and Latino communities reported higher prevalence of COVID-19 cases and COVID-19 related deaths in the past 12 months, attributed to a combination of biological and social determinants of health. That is, because these minority groups suffer disproportionately from multiple chronic health conditions and may lack access to and availability of healthcare resources, they are predisposed to the negative consequences of COVID-19. Individuals in these minority groups not only demonstrate the biological precursors to more severe outcomes resulting from COVID-19 infection, but they are also more likely to be socioeconomically disadvantaged and to have low levels of health literacy.

Compounding low levels of health literacy about vaccines in general and in combination with specific health measures such as masking, social distancing, and personal hygienic behaviors has been the barrage of misinformation delivered by trusted individuals – heads of state and news agencies. According to Kennedy (2020), "Vaccine hesitancy appears to be one aspect of a broader breakdown in trust between some sections of the population on the one hand, and elites and experts on the other." The mixed messages, recommendations, and interpretations of the data among various sources of information has led to states of confusion, indecisiveness, and disempowerment for many. Indeed, one of the greatest challenges pursuant to the pandemic will be re-establishing trust in public health authorities, locally and globally. Further, social media has provided a large-scale medium for sharing misinformation, communicating anti-vaccination sentiments, and engaging in fear mongering. Fortunately, internet technology and mass media can also communicate corrective information to targeted groups in ways that effectively counter propaganda. Together, these factors can be considered major impediments to establishing the necessary measures to control the spread of the COVID-19 virus in many communities. Addressing health illiteracy, mistrust in health authorities, and the spread of misinformation will be the work of the next generation of scientists and leaders in public health.

5.5 On the Consequences of Health *Illiteracy*

While vaccine hesitancy may represent one outcome attributable to low health literacy, it is merely one example of how health literacy or lack thereof can impact the health of individuals, communities, and populations. Other health outcomes predicted by a lack of understanding about controlling specific negative states of health or, conversely, about maintaining positive states of health include increased use of emergency health services and increased risk for hospitalization, both of which can augment healthcare costs. In the same manner, engagement with preventative health services, such as immunization programs and cancer screening programs, appear to be lower among low-health-literacy groups (Berkman et al., 2011). Health (il)literacy also occurs at the population level, encouraging or deterring public engagement in dialogue and programs aimed at promoting health and preventing disease.

As we have seen, improving health literacy can lead to greater personal autonomy and empowerment related to one's health, but it also has implications when it comes to creating healthier, more equitable communities. It is indisputable that health literacy is an important target for health policy and practice, yet there remain inconsistencies and unanswered questions. For instance, although the concept of health literacy has been around since the 1970s, there is no singular operational definition, conceptual framework, agreed-upon cutoff for identifying health literacy levels, or gold-standard measurement tool. While much research has been devoted to understanding the implications of health literacy on various aspects of health, including vaccine hesitancy, more work remains to be done to standardize health literacy assessments and advance health literacy interventions.

As discussed, achieving sufficient levels of health literacy depends on both the public and the system. Resultantly, health illiteracy must be addressed by targeting individual-level and community-level knowledge and competencies as well as bolstering public health communications and improving health services navigation. Mitigating the risks of health illiteracy on health outcomes will require the engagement of healthcare consumers, clinicians, researchers, and policy-makers alike.

5.5.1 Discussion Questions

1   The concept of literacy conveys more than merely the ability to read and write. Digital literacy and especially understanding artificial intelligence have become top of mind in many societies. Health illiteracy raises challenges that were addressed in this chapter. Consider the interaction between digital and health illiteracy. What may be some of the most critical challenges societies will face as they address the interaction between these two constructs?

2   As noted in this chapter, realizing that we are responsible for our health outcomes is a product of achieving higher health literacy. Being able to self-manage our conditions with the support of healthcare providers is necessary in optimizing our potential well-being. How might taking ownership of our health and well-being change our decisions related to specific health behaviors? Consider behaviors such as immunization, diet, lifestyle factors, and exercise. Consider how establishing health literacy with regard to such behaviors helps to shape our understanding of the social determinants of health.

Notes

1 Literacy for life, work, lifelong learning and education for democracy Report of the Secretary-General, 2020 (report #20–09756) URL: N2018899.pdf (un.org) retrieved November 2023.

2 According to the Conference Board of Canada, 48% of Canadians have inadequate literacy skills – www.conferenceboard.ca/hcp/provincial/education/adlt-lowlit.aspx January 19, 2021.

3 URL: Survey of Adult Skills (PIAAC) – PIAAC, the OECD's programme of assessment and analysis of adult skills accessed October 2021.

4 H.R.6791 – Artificial Intelligence Literacy Act of 2023: 118TH CONGRESS 1ST SESSION, "to amend the Digital Equity Act of 2021 to facilitate artificial intelligence literacy opportunities, and for other purposes."

5 Retrieved from Adult literacy | National Literacy Trust, January 30, 2024.

6 Retrieved from Media Release: New research shows the impact of illiteracy in England (prnewswire.co.uk) January 30, 2024.

7 From Exploratory Laparotomy | Saint Luke's Health System (saintlukeskc.org) retrieved February 1, 2024.

8 Biosimilar biologic drugs in Canada: Fact Sheet, www.canada.ca/content/dam/hc-sc/migration/hc-sc/dhp-mps/alt_formats/pdf/brgtherap/applic-demande/guides/Fact-Sheet-EN-2019-08-23.pdf (accessed January 23, 2021).

References

Abdel-Latif, M. M. M. (2020). The enigma of health literacy and COVID-19 pandemic. *Public Health*, *185*, 95–96.

Aldoory, L. (2017). The status of health literacy research in health communication and opportunities for future scholarship. *Health Communication*, *32*(2), 211–218. https://doi.org/10.1080/10410236.2015.1114065

Berkman, N. D., Sheridan, S. L., Donahue, K. E., Halpern, D. J., & Crotty, K. (2011). Low health literacy and health outcomes: An updated systematic review. *Annals of Internal Medicine*, *155*(2), 97–107.

Cano, R. L. E., & Lopera, H. D. E. (2013). Chapter 5: Introduction to T and B lymphocytes. In J. M. Anaya, Y. Shoenfeld, A. Rojas-Villarraga, et al. (Eds.), *Autoimmunity: From bench to bedside*. Bogota: El Rosario University Press. www.ncbi.nlm.nih.gov/books/NBK459471/

Černý, M. (2022). Searching for a definition of information literacy as a socially cohesive component of community: A complementarity of experts and student approach. *Social Sciences*, *11*, 235. https://doi.org/10.3390/socsci11060235

Coughlin, S. S., Vernon, M., Hatzigeorgiou, C., & George, V. (2020). Health literacy, social determinants of health, and disease prevention and control. *Journal of Environmental Health Sciences*, *6*(1), 3061.

Davis, F. D. (1989). Perceived usefulness, perceived ease of use, and user acceptance of information technology. *MIS Quarterly*, *13*(3), 319–340.

DeMarco, J., & Nystrom, M. (2010). The importance of health literacy in patient education. *Journal of Consumer Health on the Internet*, *14*(3), 294–301. https://doi.org/10.1080/15398285.2010.502021

De Serres, G., Markowski, F., Toth, E., Landry, M., Auger, D., Mercier, M., . . . Skowronski, D. M. (2013). Largest measles epidemic in North America in a decade – Quebec, Canada, 2011: Contribution of susceptibility, serendipity, and superspreading events. *The Journal of Infectious Diseases*, *207*(6), 990–998.

Ferigato, S., Fernandez, M., Amorim, M., Ambrogi, I., Fernandes, L. M. M., & Pacheco, R. (2020). The Brazilian Government's mistakes in responding to the COVID-19 pandemic. *The Lancet: Correspondence*, *396*, 1636.

Ford, E. S., Bergmann, M. M., Kröger, J., Schienkiewitz, A., Weikert, C., & Boeing, H. (2009). Healthy living is the best revenge: Findings from the European Prospective Investigation into Cancer and Nutrition-Potsdam study. *Archives of Internal Medicine*, *169*(15), 1355–1362. https://doi.org/10.1001/archinternmed.2009.237

Gangarosa, E. J., Galazka, A. M., Wolfe, C. R., Phillips, L. M., Miller, E., Chen, R. T., & Gangarosa, R. E. (1998). Impact of anti-vaccine movements on pertussis control: The untold story. *The Lancet*, *351*(9099), 356–361.

Güner, M. D., & Ekmekci, P. E. (2019). A survey study evaluating and comparing the health literacy knowledge and communication skills used by nurses and physicians. *INQUIRY: The Journal of Health Care Organization, Provision, and Financing*, *56*.

Hickey, K. T., Masterson Creber, R. M., Reading, M., Sciacca, R. R., Riga, T. C., Frulla, A. P., & Casida, J. M. (2018). Low health literacy: Implications for managing cardiac patients in practice. *Nurse Practitioner*, *43*(8), 49–55. https://doi.org/10.1097/01.NPR.0000541468.54290.49

Kennedy, J. (2020). Vaccine hesitancy: A growing concern. *Paediatr Drugs*, *22*(2), 105–111. doi:10.1007/s40272-020-00385-4

Kwan, B., Frankish, J., Rootman, I., Zumbo, B., Kelly, K., Begoray, D., . . . Hayes, M. (2006). *The development and validation of measures of "health literacy" in different populations*. UBC Institute of Health Promotion Research and University of Victoria Community Health Promotion Research.

LeBien, T. W., & Tedder, T. F. (2008). B lymphocytes: How they develop and function. *Blood*, *112*(5), 1570–1580. https://doi.org/10.1182/blood-2008-02-078071

Liu, C., Wang, D., Liu, C., Jiang, J., Wang, X., Chen, H., . . . Zhang, X. (2020). What is the meaning of health literacy? A systematic review and qualitative synthesis. *Family Medicine and Community Health*, *8*(2), e000351. https://doi.org/10.1136/fmch-2020-000351

Long, D., & Magerko, B. (2020, April). What is AI literacy? Competencies and design considerations. In *CHI '20: Proceedings of the 2020 CHI conference on human factors in computing systems* (pp. 1–16). https://doi.org/10.1145/3313831.3376727

Murray, J. (2021). Literacy is inadequate: Young children need literacies. *International Journal of Early Years Education*, *29*(1), 1–5. https://doi.org/10.1080/09669760.2021.1883816

Nielsen-Bohlman, L., Panzer, A. M., & Kindig, D. A. (Eds.) (2004). *Health literacy: A prescription to end confusion.* Washington (DC): National Academies Press (US)/Institute of Medicine (US) Committee on Health Literacy.

Nikou, S., De Reuver, M., & Mahboob Kanafi, M. (2022). Workplace literacy skills – how information and digital literacy affect adoption of digital technology. *Journal of Documentation*, *78*(7), pp. 371–391. https://doi.org/10.1108/JD-12-2021-0241

Olisarova, V., Kaas, J., Staskova, V., Bartlova, S., Papp, K., Nagorska, M., . . . Reifsnider, E. (2021). Health literacy and behavioral health factors in adults. *Public Health*, *190*, 75–81.

Paterick, T. E., Patel, N., Tajik, A. J., & Chandrasekaran, K. (2017). Improving health outcomes through patient education and partnerships with patients. *Proceedings (Baylor University. Medical Center)*, *30*(1), 112–113. https://doi.org/10.1080/08998280.2017.11929552

Prince, L., Schmidtke, C., Beck, J. K., & Hadden, K. (2018). An assessment of organizational health literacy practices at an academic health center. *Quality Management in Health Care*, *27*(2), 93–97. https://doi.org/10.1097/QMH.0000000000000162

Programme for the International Assessment of Adult Competencies. (2013). *Ministry of Industry, Canada. Skills in Canada: First results from the Programme for the International Assessment of Adult Competencies (PIAAC).* https://www150.statcan.gc.ca/n1/pub/89-555-x/89-555-x2013001-eng.pdf

Protheroe, J., Nutbeam, D., & Rowlands, G. (2009). Health literacy: A necessity for increasing participation in health care. *The British Journal of General Practice*, *59*(567), 721–723. https://doi.org/10.3399/bjgp09X472584

Schwarz, G. (2005). Overview: What is media literacy, who cares, and why? *Teachers College Record*, *107*, 13, 5–17.

Selenko, E., Bankins, S., Shoss, M., Warburton, J., & Restubog, S. L. D. (2022). Artificial intelligence and the future of work: A functional-identity perspective. *Current Directions in Psychological Science*, *31*(3), 272–279.

Simoes, E. J., & Jackson-Thompson, J. (2023). The United States public health services failure to control the coronavirus epidemic. *Preventive Medicine Reports*, *31*, 102090. https://doi.org/10.1016/j.pmedr.2022.102090

Speros, C. (2005). Health literacy: Concept analysis. *Journal of Advanced Nursing*, *50*(6), 633–640.

Stormacq, C., Wosinski, J., Boillat, E., & Van den Broucke, S. (2020). Effects of health literacy interventions on health-related outcomes in socioeconomically disadvantaged adults living in the community: A systematic review. *JBI Evidence Synthesis*, *18*(7), 1389–1469. https://doi.org/10.11124/JBISRIR-D-18-00023

Tai, D. B. G., Shah, A., Doubeni, C. A., Sia, I. G., & Wieland, M. L. (2021). The disproportionate impact of COVID-19 on racial and ethnic minorities in the United States. *Clinical Infectious Diseases*, *72*(4), 703–706.

Tinmaz, H., Lee, Y. T., Fanea-Ivanovici, M., & Baber, H. (2022). A systematic review on digital literacy. *Smart Learning Environments*, *9*, 21. https://doi.org/10.1186/s40561-022-00204-y

Vikram, K., Vanneman, R., & Desai, S. (2012). Linkages between maternal education and childhood immunization in India. *Social Science & Medicine*, *75*(2), 331–339.

Zegers, C. A., Gonzales, K., Smith, L. M., Pullen, C. H., De Alba, A., & Fiandt, K. (2020). The psychometric testing of the functional, communicative, and critical health literacy tool. *Patient Education and Counseling*, *103*(11), 2347–2352.

The Microbiome and How Your Food Choices Affect Your Health

6.0 Introduction

When we think of microorganisms, most of us think of nasty germs that make us ill.

However, not all bugs are bad!

In fact, many microorganisms support our daily physiological functions along with the mental and physical health of our body (Gilbert et al., 2018). The human *microbiota*, a term used to describe the multitude of organisms inhabiting our body (Grice and Segre, 2011; Cresci and Bawden, 2015; Santacroce et al., 2020), can exhibit a variety of relationships: organisms can be commensal, meaning they feed off of us without causing harm; mutualistic, meaning that there is a shared symbiotic relationship in which each organism gains benefits because of the presence of each other; or pathogenic, meaning they cause harm or disease to the host. In other words, they make you and me sick (Ogunrinola et al., 2020)!

6.0.1 Important Background

In the biosphere, we classify living creatures using a hierarchical system, a taxonomy, that begins at the top with domains and then progresses down through kingdom, phylum, class, order, family, genus, species, and in some instances, we may even report variety. When we describe the biosphere, we are most often referring to the living organisms that make up the inhabitants of our planet. Each living organism follows a blueprint throughout its lifespan dictated by a sequence of genetic information – a genome – in the form of DNA (deoxyribonucleic acid) or RNA (ribonucleic acid). Each molecule, DNA and RNA, is a nucleic acid made up of building blocks known as nucleotides. Nucleotides are made up of three subunits (combinations of molecules): a nitrogenous base, a sugar, and phosphate. The four nitrogenous bases that constitute a molecule of DNA are (A) adenine, (T) thymine, (C) cytosine, and (G) guanine. The bases can be categorized into two groups: purines and pyrimidines. Molecules of adenine and guanine have a distinct double-ring structure consisting of a hexagonal pyrimidine ring and a

DOI: 10.4324/9781003474777-6

pentagonal imidazole ring which, together, combine to form a purine. The molecules of cytosine and thymine are single-ring hexagonal structures known as pyrimidines. In RNA, the nitrogenous base thymine is replaced with the nitrogenous base uracil, which is also a single-ring pyrimidine.

DNA is often called the blueprint of life because the instructional information for how we grow and develop is presented in its structure and arrangement of nucleotides. Although both DNA and RNA consist of nucleotides, they differ in structure and in function. The nucleotides in a molecule of DNA are arranged as a double-strand helix of nucleotides connected at the bases to form base pairs. In DNA, the base pairs consist of adenine and thymine as one connection and cytosine and guanine as the other connecting base pair.

In RNA, nucleotides are arranged in a single strand, with the sugar molecule comprising each nucleotide being a ribose (having an OH on the #2 carbon), in contrast to DNA, in which the sugar is deoxyribose (having H on the #2 carbon). Hence the names ribonucleic acid (RNA) and deoxyribonucleic acid (DNA). Although there is no base-pair connection in the single strand of RNA, the arrangement of the nucleotides in RNA is important for transcribing genetic information to direct the synthesis of amino acids that are the building blocks of protein structures.

6.0.2 Ribosomes and Protein Synthesis

Proteins are essential to our existence because they have many roles throughout our lifespan. Proteins not only form structures such as bones, skin, cartilage, muscles, and vessels, they also have storage functions (ferritin for iron storage), contractile functions (in skeletal, smooth, and cardiac muscle contraction – actin and myosin), receptor functions (visual proteins – rhodopsin), transport functions (oxygen transport – hemoglobin and myoglobin), protective functions (immunoglobulin), hormonal functions (insulin), and catalyst functions, because all enzymes are proteins. Proteins are formed from amino acids connected in a linear arrangement, where the amino acids are the building blocks – aka fundamental structures required to produce proteins.

Within the cytosol, there exist special organelles called ribosomes that are essential to the synthesis of proteins through the process of translation (Opron and Burton, 2019). Ribosomes can be in the cytoplasm or attached to the rough endoplasmic reticulum (RER), the sub-structure of the endoplasmic reticulum (ER), which is located adjacent to the cell's nucleus and which functions in protein synthesis but is dependent on the destination of the specific proteins that are produced (Sanvictores and Davis, 2023).

Ribosomes are composed of a ribosomal RNA (rRNA) and protein organized into two sub-units: large or small. Protein synthesis involves three main components: ribosomal RNA, which forms the structure of the ribosome and gives rise to its function; transfer RNA, which is the molecule that transfers the transcribed DNA information into amino acids for protein synthesis; and messenger RNA, which is responsible for transcribing the DNA information in the nucleus and carrying the information to the ribosome in the cytosol for interaction with transfer RNA (Zhou et al., 2015). Together, these three mechanisms transfer the essential pattern of information for protein creation (synthesis) from RNA nucleotides to amino acids, which eventually form the longer chains of protein. Although highly complicated, the process of nucleotide transfer to protein is explained in simple terms here.

We begin with a strand of messenger RNA (mRNA).[1] This strand holds nucleotides arranged in groups of three called codons. The plan for arranging the nucleotides into the tri-nucleotide codon occurs in a cell's nucleus and is a process known as transcription. During transcription, the pattern of nucleotides is copied from the DNA to the mRNA and then transported from the nucleus to the cytosol, where the ribosomes are located. The mRNA then enters a ribosome, where it interacts with a highly specific and highly selective transfer RNA (tRNA) carrying an amino acid. The correct tRNA connects to the complementary base of the codon (trinucleotide) on the mRNA molecule to deliver the corresponding amino acid and form the building blocks of protein.

We can think of the ribosomal mRNA-to-tRNA transfer process like a train (mRNA) carrying specific passengers (codons) that have friends (tRNA) waiting to pick them up at the station (ribosomal RNA). When mRNA arrives at the station with a codon that has, for example, the bases organized as adenine-guanine-uracil, then the tRNA that would show up to retrieve this specific codon and the tRNA structure would be arranged as the complementary to the codon, called an anticodon, so that the bases would be organized as uracil-cytosine-adenine. By carrying the complementary set of bases, the tRNA can bind to this codon to enable translation to occur as the next step in amino acid formation. Subsequently, by stringing amino acids together in a linear arrangement, we begin to create or synthesize specific proteins – hence the process of protein synthesis.

6.1 The Domains

In 1990, Wheelis, Kandler, and Woese introduced the reorganization of the taxonomy of living creatures based not on overtly observable characteristics, such as presence of dimples or scales versus skin, fins versus ambulatory appendages, or egg-hatched versus live birth but on the molecular relationships between living creatures (Wheelis et al., 1992). More specifically, they used differences in the ribosomal RNA structures to create the classification table of creatures within specific groups. Using ribosomal RNA (rRNA) as a categorizing strategy, Wheelis and coworkers proposed that the biological system of classification should produce three super-kingdoms – the domains. These three domains are (i) bacteria, (ii) archaea, and (iii) eukarya.

Humans are part of the third domain – the eukarya – and as such, we share the same ribosomal RNA as a fruit fly, but our ribosomal RNA is different from that of bacteria.

The domains of bacteria and archaea belong to the cell classification of prokaryotes, while the cells in the domain of eukarya are classified as eukaryotes. These two main cell classifications – prokaryotes and eukaryotes – are distinguished from each other by the elements within each domain's cytosol (the fluid part within the cell). Notably, prokaryotes are unicellular, while eukaryotes can be unicellular (e.g., yeast) or multicellular.

However, as we continue to develop more sophisticated analytical methods, we are challenging the dogma that once described the characteristics that differentiated prokaryotes from eukaryotes. Previously, it was believed that prokaryotes were simple cells with no organelle structures to encase the machinery of cell function. However, recent research has shown that prokaryotes have distinct compartments within the cytosol that enable selected cell machinery to provide specific functions (Murat et al., 2010).

Following continued exploration of the structure of prokaryotic cells, we are learning that the elements of the prokaryote cytosol compartments can be both unique in form and highly specific in functionality. For example, in a type of prokaryotic bacteria known as *magnetotactic bacteria*, researchers have shown the presence of magnetosomes (Lefèvre and Bazylinski, 2013), which are structures that help the cells to physically orient themselves within magnetic fields, which, in turn, enables bacteria to carry out selective cell functioning.

Although prokaryotes and eukaryotes are mostly distinct in structure and function, there are similarities in both the constituents and the functions of the cells across the two domains. For example, ribosomes, which carry out protein synthesis in eukaryotic cells, are also found in the cytosol of prokaryotes, and each ribosomal molecule includes both ribosomal proteins (mRNA and tRNA) and is made from ribosomal RNA that together perform selective functions (Murat et al., 2010).

The eukarya, or eukaryote cells, is the classification group to which both we humans and fungi – the mushrooms in your salad – belong. Eukarya has nuclei and membrane-bound structures that provide specific functions distinct from those of the prokaryotic cells (Fuerst, 2010). The nuclei and mitochondria are examples of two elements we see within a eukaryotic cell that are not present in prokaryote cells.

The nuclei, which may have first been described by van Leeuwenhoek (Pederson, 2011) in 1710 or by Brown in 1830 (Lamond and Earnshaw, 1998), are an essential constituent of the eukaryotic cell that is not found in prokaryotic cells (Cooper, 2000). The nuclei are in the cytosol – the fluid part of the cytoplasm. They function both as the storehouse of cellular genetic material (the nucleic acids) in the form of chromosomes – deoxyribonucleic acid (DNA) and ribonucleic acid (RNA) – and as the site where DNA and RNA processing occurs.

Another source of genomic material important to our discussion of the microbiome is the DNA of the mitochondria (Franco-Obregón and Gilbert, 2017). Mitochondrial DNA (mtDNA) is much smaller and simpler than nuclear DNA and holds only 16,569 pairs of the adenine (A), cytosine (C), guanine (G), and thymine (T) (AGCT) bases (Wright and Bottino, 1986). Unlike mitochondrial DNA, nuclear DNA has some 3 billion base pairs (Brown, 2002), and although the base pairs of DNA in the mitochondria are the same compounds as those of the DNA in the nuclei, the double-stranded alpha-helix structure of mitochondrial DNA is arranged as a circular chromosome rather than as a linear structure.

The mitochondria in the cell's cytosol provide important cell functions. The main role of mitochondrial DNA is to produce the functional parts within the mitochondria that lead to energy production. Mitochondria are essential to eukaryotic cells because they hold the machinery that leads to aerobic (oxygen-based) energy production. Often described as the powerhouse of the cell, mitochondria can produce energy in the form of adenosine triphosphate (ATP) through the oxidative energy transfer processes for fats and carbohydrates. For example, the simple anaerobic energy transfer process of glycolytic metabolism is enhanced 18-fold when moving from anaerobic glycolysis to the oxidative processes of the tricarboxylic acid cycle (aka the Krebs Cycle) and the electron transport chain.

Additionally, while mitochondria provide energy upon which life and activity are possible, they are also contributors to the natural cycle of death in eukaryote cells through the process known as apoptosis (Green and Reed, 1998). On a positive note, all mitochondria are provided by your mother, and therefore, mitochondrial DNA can be used to trace your maternal ancestry.

6.2 The Microbiome

Although as humans, we believe ourselves to be unique members of the domain of eukaryotes, we thrive in our ecological space directly connected to other eukarya, bacteria, and archaea. In fact, while we assume that we are independent autonomous creatures inhabiting the planet Earth, we exist in the shared space of the biosphere (Pace, 1997; Cryan et al., 2019), not as independent entities but as transport vehicles for other eukarya, bacteria, and archaea in a community that we refer to as the microbiome.

The term *microbiome* refers to the group of microscopic organisms – which cannot be seen with our naked eye – but which live on and inside our bodies. These microorganisms represent each of the three domains of the biological classification hierarchy. That is, the microbiome includes bacteria, archaea, and eukarya, and is often measured by the proportions of bacteria, viruses, fungi, and protozoa that constitute all elements in the microbiome. The term *microbiota* is used to describe the entire colony of undifferentiated constituents that make up the microbiome. Frequently, the terms *microbiome* and *microbiota* are considered synonymous and can be used interchangeably.

Viruses, which are included as constituents of the microbiome, are neither prokaryotes nor eukaryotes because they do not contain cells and lack the ability to replicate without a host (Louten, 2016). A virus is an obligate intracellular parasite consisting of genetic material, either as DNA or RNA, encapsulated by a protein coat called a capsid. Interestingly, the structure of viruses and their ability to replicate via the process of transcription when reliant on a host perpetuates the conversation about whether viruses are alive or dead. However, according to Koonin and Starokadomskyy, 2016), the better contribution to knowledge of viruses is not to debate whether they are living or dead but rather to consider viruses relative to their functional actions. That is, given that viruses are replicators, viruses should be considered as mechanisms, and therefore, we need to determine whether the mechanistic action of the virus is that of being either a selfish replicator like a plasmid or as a cooperative replicator like a chromosome.

Yet regardless of where viruses occur on the selfishness-to-cooperativity spectrum, they are part of our microbiome (Abeles and Pride, 2014; Handley, 2016) because they co-exist with the bacteria and eukarya of our microbiome. Moreover, bacteria and eukarya function as the host constituent for the virus to function. Viruses are structures that transport genetic material in the form of a double-stranded helix of DNA (dsDNA), single strands of DNA (sDNA), double strands of RNA (dsRNA), or single strands of RNA (ssRNA). As described by Louten, viruses are composed of nucleic acids surrounded by a capsid – a structure of repeating proteins that encircles the nucleic acid strands. The capsid–nucleic acid complex can be protected by an external lipid layer to form an enveloped virus, or it can exist without a protective lipid envelope, which gives rise to a naked virus. In both the enveloped virus and the naked virus, there are attachment proteins in the capsid layer that enable the virus to attach to receptors on the surface of a host cell. A recent star in the realm of viruses is that which the world has come to know as the SARS CoV-2 virus, the main attraction in our recent COVID-19 pandemic. SARS CoV-2 virus is an enveloped single-stranded RNA (ssRNA) virus which has spike projections on the viral envelope that enable the virus to attach to host cells. The positioning of the projecting spike proteins gives the appearance of a crown-like capsid structure, which is why it is labelled a coronavirus (Li, 2016).

Note that in this discussion, we mentioned the capsid, which is the protein coat that encases the genetic material (ssRNA). This envelope is a lipid membrane that surrounds the capsid and forms the outermost layer. This outer layer contains the attachment or spike proteins. Enveloped viruses are more fragile than naked viruses because the lipid bilayer membrane is more susceptible to damage by heat, pH changes, detergent, and environmental conditions – e.g., dry environments, toxic stimuli in the environment.

6.3 What Is the Role of the Microbiome?

Each of us is a biosphere in that our physical mass is harboring and nurturing multiple ecosystems that are in a constant state of flux. The microorganisms that comprise our microbiome co-exist in a symbiotic relationship with humans. More specifically, we humans are coated by trillions of these microscopic creatures, both on and inside our bodies, with multiple different types of microbiota communities in the different parts of our bodies. Previous research by Ursel and coworkers (2012) suggests that we transport some 100 trillion of these commensal creatures within our gut microbiome. Interestingly, although it has been suggested that our human body cells, or soma, are outnumbered by the microorganisms of the microbiome by a factor of at least 10:1, research by Sender et al. (2016) indicated that the real ratio may be considerably less given the amount of variation across humans, and according to their estimates, the bacteria-to-human-cell ratio may even be closer to 1:1.

As noted by Cryan and coworkers (2019), the diversity of microorganisms that are distributed across our bodies is an evolving process throughout our lifespan. While we begin with the initial microbiota of the birthing process, our activities and exposures during our lives contribute to our microbiome. As we age, we observe that stress, diet, environment, and lifestyle each contribute to the characteristics, type, volume, and diversity of our microbiome.

As we continue to learn about the microbiome, we are discovering most of its functions are commensal, meaning that the microorganisms which use our body as the host do so without affecting us negatively. The microbiome has been linked to the production of important resources through the bioconversion of nutrients as well as in protecting against pathogenic microbes. As a biosphere, our various physiological systems – which include, for example, our immune system (Dietert and Dietert, 2012), our cardiovascular system (Ahmed and Spence, 2021), and our gut-to-brain axis (Cryan et al., 2019) – work in concert with our microbiome to prevent diseases by fighting off invading pathogens, the naughty microbes that would do us harm. In effect, many of the microorganisms that constitute the microbiota of the microbiome may even have a positive role in our existence and be supportive of our physical, mental, and emotional health in what can be considered a mutualistic (or mutually beneficial) relationship with *YOU*!

Yes, you! Research by Fierer and colleagues (2010) showed that using sensitive pyrosequencing techniques to detect gene sequences, the researchers could match the unique genetic information from an individual's skin surface with the genetic information left behind on their keyboards from the microbiome of their skin. This research is important because it shows that with the right equipment that has the appropriate sensitivity and specificity, there is a real opportunity to discern an individual based on their microbiota.

Where do we find the microbiome, and where do all these bugs come from?

The microorganism constituents of the microbiome are located across our entire body. For example, microbiota have been identified on our skin and mucous membranes, in our upper respiratory and gastrointestinal tracts, on the outer opening of the urethra, on the external surfaces of our genitalia, in the vagina, in the external ear canal, and on the external surface of the eyelids and in the conjunctiva, the mucous membrane that covers the eye and inner surface of the eyelids.

The human microbiome is acquired from the environment in each successive generation. As infants, we receive our initial dose of microbiota during the birthing process as we pass through our mother's vagina. Several researchers have reported that the mode of birth (i.e., conventional vaginal delivery versus Caesarean section) can influence the type and volume of microbiota on an infant (Sokolowska et al., 2018; Lemas et al., 2016; Ursell et al., 2012). According to Ursell et al. (2012), the infant's microbiome, when delivered by conventional vaginal birth, can resemble that of the mother's vagina within 20 minutes after birth, while children born by Caesarean section have a microbiome profile that reflects that which is found on the mother's skin. However, as Manson et al. (2008) reported, the gut microbiome is in a constant state of flux so that the community of bacteria, archaea, eukaryotes, and viruses is consistently changing.

Most notably, during the early stages of a child's development, there will be an ongoing establishment of bacteria within the microbiome, and this environment will be continuously changing as a function of age and diet. For example, Lemas et al. (2016) reported that development of the infant gut microbiome is influenced by several factors that include not only genetics and mode of delivery but also whether the child was breastfed or formula fed. In particular, the researchers noted that the gut microbiome of the infant results from the dynamic exchange between the mother and the child early in life. Perinatal development – that period of time during gestation and up to one year following birth – is a period when the child's microbiome is characteristic of the developmental environment of the womb and includes maternal blood supply, amniotic fluid, and meconium (the infant's first post-partum bowel movement) (Lemas et al., 2016). During and following delivery, the infant's microbiome is rapidly influenced by birth mode as well as by skin-to-skin contact and feeding modality (i.e., breastfed or formula fed).

As an essential prophylactic, the microbiome will have a direct influence on the human immune system and will thereby assist in providing resistance to the development of specific diseases. According to Sokolowska and coworkers, within the gut microbiota, dysbiosis that results from poor development of the microbiome is associated with an increased risk of developing allergies and asthma later in life. Earlier research suggested that a reduction in our microbiome and especially a loss of *microbiota diversity* – the measure of how many different species of microorganisms make up our microbiome – is linked to autoimmune diseases and obesity as well as cardio-metabolic conditions. Microbiome diversity indices are often used to quantify the distribution of microbiota in our microbiome but may be of limited value because the indices cannot provide information about composition and function (Johnson and Burnet, 2016). However, as noted by Johnson and Burnet (2016), having a diverse microbiome may be an indicator of a stable microbiome.

In a later review by Cullen and coworkers (2020), the authors reported that individuals that ingest a prescribed regimen of antimicrobials can reduce their microbiota diversity, which, in turn, can lead to dysbiosis (aka: microbial imbalance) that may require a prolonged time for recovery. During this period of dysbiosis, the microbiome can have a disrupted composition and function that can increase the risk of being infected by pathogenic microbes that would otherwise be restricted by a more diverse microbiota.

6.4 On the Importance of the Gut Microbiome and Chronic Disease

Our understanding of the importance of gut microbiota is relatively recent and is constantly emerging. Research on the indigenous microbial communities, meaning original microbial communities that make up the microbiome, is a result of our ability to evaluate the constituents using relatively recent developments in genomic methods such as high-throughput DNA sequencing techniques (Weinstock, 2012). Manson et al. (2008) and Su et al. (2012) described the use of culture-independent techniques, which focus on measuring the small sub-unit ribosomal RNA gene as having enhanced our ability to evaluate the microbiome and the host environment that they inhabit. According to Cocolin and colleagues (2013), the use of culture-independent techniques, which were initially developed to evaluate food fermentation, have since led to a deeper understanding of microbiome diversity and thereby have enhanced the evolution of our knowledge and changed clinicians' ideas about the importance of microbes in human health and disease processes. The notion that microbiomes are useful for human health is only part of the understanding that has helped to enhance our knowledge. More important is the realization that most of the microbiota that exist on or in our body are providing beneficial outcomes for the entire host–microbe system (Young, 2017).

The relationship between the gut microbiome and chronic disease is well established (Pascal et al., 2018; Madhogaria et al., 2022). Cancer, obesity, inflammatory bowel disease, and cardiovascular disease seem to be the most thoroughly studied to date because of the ability to identify and measure two specific bacterial groups in the microbiome: (i) the firmicutes and (ii) the bacteroidetes. The firmicutes are classified as gram-positive bacteria, which means that they do not have an outer tunic or membrane coating and thereby are more likely to absorb elements in their environment; hence the reason that they stain positive (purple dye in the gram stain test). The bacteroidetes are classified as gram-negative bacteria and differ from firmicutes in that they have a thick lipid tunic, or outer membrane that makes them less permeable to absorbing chemicals in their environment. The gram-negative bacteroidetes stain pink because they do not absorb the gram stain during testing.

Together, the firmicutes and bacteroidetes of the microbiome comprise some 90% of the microbiota (Magne et al., 2020) and help to support the physical health of the host through specific biosynthesis activities in the gut. For example, Singh et al. (2017)

described the importance of the gut microbiome for vitamin production and production of essential amino acids (Singh et al., 2017). Recent research on diet and the development of the microbiome has shown that even acute changes in diet can have a measurable effect on the composition and distribution of gut microbiota. For example, plant-based diets lead to outcomes that are different than animal-based diets, especially concerning the presence of firmicutes and bacteroidetes. Similarly, diets having high volumes of sugar have a different influence again on the colonization and distribution of microbes within the gut microbiome (Magne et al., 2020).

According to Magne and coworkers (2020), an important biomarker of dysbiosis in the gut microbiome is the firmicutes-to-bacteroidetes ratio (F/B), which is believed to be influenced by nutrient consumption (Garcia-Mantrana et al., 2018). More specifically, a higher ratio score for firmicutes to bacteroidetes appears to be associated with a higher prevalence of chronic diseases. However, while this potential link seems promising, much more research needs to be done to partition out the possible confounding effects of lifestyle behaviors and environmental contaminants. For example, while Garcia-Mantrana and coworkers showed that individuals who consumed more animal protein, saturated fat, and sugars had lower gut microbiota diversity and a higher F/B ratio, the sample was based on a group of healthy volunteers ($N = 27$, 16 females and 11 males) with a mean age of 39.5 years who were living in a Mediterranean region of Spain. The authors suggested that there may be a link between type of nutrient consumption and increased risk of chronic disease, but such small studies need to be critically reviewed and replicated before omnibus generalizations can be established.

Ongoing research in this area continues to show important relationships between the gut microbiome and physical, mental, and emotional health because of the type of nutrients we consume. According to Jamar et al. (2021), there are distinct differences in the gut microbiome response that are related to microbe diversity and neurophysiological functioning associated with differences in diets. Most notably, diets high in monosaturated fats will have different effects on gut microbiota when compared to diets high in saturated fats and to diets high in sugars (most often sucrose-based sugars). For example, as Zinöcker and Lindseth (2018) suggested, the Western diet, which is the typical North American diet, being high in fats and sugars, is extremely detrimental because sugars and fats have a direct influence on promoting inflammatory mechanisms.

6.5 Diet and the Microbiome

At this point, we understand that multiple factors affect the microbiome, not the least of which are diet, environmental contaminants, epigenetics, stress, and lifestyle. How do we make positive changes that can help our microbiome and enhance our ability to achieve positive states of physical, mental, and emotional health?

From a North American perspective, our earlier approach to nutrient consumption was to avoid fat. That is, we became obsessed about overall fat, suggesting that no more than 30% of our daily caloric intake be made up of fat and no more than 10% of our caloric intake be made up of saturated fats and only 10% of polyunsaturated fats (Krauss et al., 1996). However, as we continue to develop our knowledge about the microbiome, we are changing our messages about nutrient consumption, energy balance, and the ability to control our risks of chronic disease in an intentional way.

In the developed world that includes countries from the G20, such as the United States, Canada, the U.K., and the Scandinavian countries, for example, food type is far more important than caloric consumption. In the developing world and in the world of people displaced because of catastrophic upheaval – wars and the inability to recover from natural disasters – caloric consumption and famine are existential issues that have a severe impact on the microbiome. The macronutrients (fats, carbohydrates, and protein) are essential to the discussion. However, in understanding the important role of the microbiome in our health, we need to recognize the factors that have both a direct and indirect influence on its potential function.

Without question, the microbiome is influenced by the type of processed foods we eat, the volumes of chlorinated and contaminated water we drink, the influence of stressors – physical, psychological, emotional – to which we are exposed during our early years of development, and the implicit and explicit behaviors of our lifestyle, some of which include substance use, exercise, and relaxation/coping strategies (Zinöcker and Lindseth, 2018). Research supports our perspective that the gut microbiome is directly associated with our health because it protects against opportunistic pathogens, contributes to the management of our immune system functions, enables digestion of foodstuffs, leading to biosynthesis of vitamins and essential amino acids, and contributes to the production and balance of energy to perform work through metabolism. Moreover, microbiota regulate the metabolic functions of the host (that's us!) and can contribute to both synthetic and catabolic effects through direct host-to-microbe interactions.

Yet we also know that foods can harm the microbiome (Zinöcker and Lindseth, 2018), creating the condition we call dysbiosis (Chen et al., 2023), and therefore, we need to increase our awareness of what constitutes a positive microbiome community (Rinninella et al., 2019). Fried foods, most notably the deep-fried variety, are of concern because frying oil triggers a series of chemical changes that increase the concentrations of trans-fatty acids while decreasing the concentration of polyunsaturated fats (Qi, 2021). Likewise, consumption of sugar, especially refined white sugar, is becoming recognized more frequently as a negatively influential food source for the microbiome, but sugar in any form has the potential to impact your gut health (Di Rienzi and Britton, 2020). Therefore, we need to be critical consumers; we need to read labels and take note of the proportions of the chemicals that can cause us physiological harm directly, like the glucose-to-fructose ratio. For example, Townsend et al. (2019) reported that a diet rich in fructose can influence your gut microbiome by preventing the beneficial microbiota from colonizing in the gut. Preventing colonization of good microbiota can inhibit the production of specific proteins that support continued propagation of beneficial bacterial species.

In a comprehensive review of the role of diet quality and the type of nutrient intake, Hills et al. (2019) described the negative consequences of the Western diet, the typical diet for the North American population, in which sugar, fats and processed foods are extensively promoted through various forms of media. Hills reported that the North American diet is implicated in the loss of microbiome diversity and, as a result, a loss in the microbiome's diverse functionality. Hills and colleagues presented research evidence of the associated negative consequences of losing diversity in the microbiome on physical and mental health.

The loss or reduction in propagation of good bacteria such as the firmicutes and bacteroidetes, which assist in processing complex carbohydrates, and the production of short-chain fatty acids (SCFA) is extremely important to maintaining good gut health (Hills et al., 2019; Tan et al., 2014; Pan et al., 2009). The production of SCFA is an essential metabolic end product from the process of gut fermentation of non-digested carbohydrates (Portincasa et al., 2022; Morrison and Preston, 2016). SCFAs are used in energy production and changing pH within the GI tract that reduces the likelihood of pathogen growth and enhances absorption and excretion (Oh et al., 2019; Morrison and Preston, 2016).

Likewise, because SCFAs can cross the blood–brain barrier (Silva et al., 2020), they appear to be involved in the promotion of neural regeneration and are prevalent as important players in the communication pathway between the gut and the brain known as the gut–microbiota–brain axis. Increased production of SCFAs from the consumption of dietary fiber leading to fermentation of the prebiotics galactooligosaccharides (GOS), fructooligosaccharides (FOS), and the polysaccharide inulin (Hills et al., 2019), which result from hydrolysis of complex carbohydrates, are also linked to glycemic control, satiety, and subsequent weight loss.

However, to accomplish the proposed outcomes identified in the research reported here, we need to start with the appropriate diet. As noted, the Western diet is not the appropriate choice to enable us to gain the benefits of microbiome function (Myles, 2014). As Hills and coworkers reported, within immigrant cohorts that consumed the Western diet, the obesity risk showed a fourfold increase within 15 years of immigrating to the USA, in comparison to what it would have been had they stayed in their own country. Conversely, the Mediterranean diet has been associated with the consumption of appropriate foods that enhance the diversity and function of the microbiome, leading to positive physical and mental health gains.

6.6 Conclusion

The genetic diversity found within our gut microbiota is important in the proliferation of chronic disease. Among the more studied areas, we understand that our microbiome changes in response to what we eat. As noted, consumption of fiber-rich and fermented foods enhances the production of prebiotics, which promotes colonies of beneficial bacteria. Conversely, if our diet consists of the typical North American fast food, packaged snacks, and frozen meals laden with harmful ingredients, our microbiome will respond with an overgrowth of unfriendly microbes.

The gut microbiome is a community of life-forms that has tremendous potential to either support us or end us! Moreover, humans in the developed world can control the communities of microbiota that will colonize the gut. But individuals in developing countries that are predominantly food insecure are at a greater risk of gut dysbiosis because of the quality and quantity of foodstuffs that are considered of low nutritional value.

As we learn more about the microbiome, we see the direct link between microbiome dysbiosis and developmental issues that have epigenetic effects based on phenotypic outcomes caused by environments such as food insecurity. Likewise, as we investigate the microbiome in the affluent world, we realize how our lifestyle has a direct and often negative impact on our food choices and the unwitting harm we are doing to our gut microbiome and other systems of the body.

6.6.1 Discussion Questions

1 As noted in this chapter, we are not alone! Our bodies contain trillions of microorganisms that assist our development throughout our lifespan. Consider how the microbiome is essential for our health from a physical and mental health perspective.

2 Considering that the human microbiome is acquired from the environment, how do the social determinants of health influence the development of our microbiome and contribute to our overall health and well-being?

Note

1 mRNA serves as a template and carries genetic information from DNA in codons. tRNA carries specific amino acids and has an anticodon region that recognizes and forms base pairs with the codon on mRNA. tRNA transfers the amino acids in a linear sequence guided by mRNA to form a polypeptide chain – a protein.

References

Abeles SR, Pride DT. Molecular bases and role of viruses in the human microbiome. *J Mol Biol.* 2014;426(23):3892–3906. doi:10.1016/j.jmb.2014.07.002

Ahmed S, Spence JD. Sex differences in the intestinal microbiome: Interactions with risk factors for atherosclerosis and cardiovascular disease. *Biol Sex Differ.* 2021;12:35. doi:10.1186/s13293-021-00378-z

Brown, TA. Chapter 1: The human genome. In *Genomes.* 2nd edition. Oxford: Wiley-Liss; 2002.

Chen J, Xiao Y, Li D, Zhang S, Wu Y, Zhang Q, Bai W. New insights into the mechanisms of high-fat diet mediated gut microbiota in chronic diseases. *iMeta.* 2023;2:e69. doi:10.1002/imt2.69

Cocolin L, Alessandria V, Dolci P, Gorra R, Rantsiou K. Culture independent methods to assess the diversity and dynamics of microbiota during food fermentation. *Int J Food Microbiol.* 2013;167(1):29–43. doi:10.1016/j.ijfoodmicro.2013.05.008

Cooper GM. Chapter 8: The nucleus. In *The Cell: A Molecular Approach.* 2nd edition. Sunderland, MA: Sinauer Associates; 2000. www.ncbi.nlm.nih.gov/books/NBK9845/

Cresci GA, Bawden E. Gut microbiome: What we do and don't know. *Nutr Clin Pract.* 2015;30(6):734–746. doi:10.1177/0884533615609899

Cryan JF, O'Riordan KJ, Cowan CSM, et al. The microbiota-gut-brain axis. *Physiol Rev.* 2019;99(4):1877–2013. doi:10.1152/physrev.00018.2018

Cullen CM, Aneja KK, Beyhan S, Cho CE, Woloszynek S, Convertino M, McCoy SJ, Zhang Y, Anderson MZ, Alvarez-Ponce D, Smirnova E, Karstens L, Dorrestein PC, Li H, Sen Gupta A, Cheung K, Powers JG, Zhao Z, Rosen GL. Emerging priorities for microbiome research. *Front Microbiol.* 2020;11:136. doi:10.3389/fmicb.2020.00136

Di Rienzi SC, Britton RA. Adaptation of the gut microbiota to modern dietary sugars and sweeteners. *Adv Nutrit.* 2020;11(3):616–629. doi:10.1093/advances/nmz118

Fierer N, Lauber CL, Zhou N, McDonald D, Costello EK, Knight R. Forensic identification using skin bacterial communities. *Proc Nat Acad Sci.* 2010;107(14):6477–6481. doi:10.1073/pnas.1000162107

Franco-Obregón A, Gilbert JA. The microbiome-mitochondrion connection: Common ancestries, common mechanisms, common goals. *mSystems.* 2017;2(3):e00018. doi:10.1128/mSystems.00018-17

Fuerst JA. Beyond prokaryotes and eukaryotes: Planctomycetes and cell organization. *Nat Educ.* 2010;3(9):44.

Garcia-Mantrana I, Selma-Royo M, Alcantara C, Collado MC. Shifts on gut microbiota associated to Mediterranean diet adherence and specific dietary intakes on general adult population. *Front Microbiol.* 2018;9:890. doi:10.3389/fmicb.2018.00890

Gilbert JA, Blaser MJ, Caporaso JG, Jansson JK, Lynch SV, Knight R. Current understanding of the human microbiome. *Nat Med.* 2018;24(4):392–400. doi:10.1038/nm.4517

Green DR, Reed JC. Mitochondria and apoptosis. *Science.* 1998;281:1309–1312. doi:10.1126/science.281.5381.1309

Grice EA, Segre JA. The skin microbiome. *Nat Rev Microbiol.* 2011;9(4):244–253.

Handley SA. The virome: A missing component of biological interaction networks in health and disease. *Genome Med.* 2016;8:32. doi:10.1186/s13073-016-0287-y

Hills RD, Pontefract BA, Mishcon HR, Black CA, Sutton SC, Theberge CR. Gut microbiome: Profound implications for diet and disease. *Nutrients.* 2019;11(7):1613. doi:10.3390/nu11071613

Jamar G, Ribeiro DA, Pisani LP. High-fat or high-sugar diets trigger inflammation in the microbiota-gut-brain axis. *Crit Rev Food Sci Nutr.* 2021;61(5):836–854. doi:10.1080/10408398.2020.1747046

Johnson KV, Burnet PW. Microbiome: Should we diversify from diversity? *Gut Microbes.* 2016;7(6):455–458. doi:10.1080/19490976.2016.1241933

Koonin EV, Starokadomskyy P. Are viruses alive? The replicator paradigm sheds decisive light on an old but misguided question. *Stud Hist Phil Sci C.* 2016;59:125–134. doi:10.1016/j.shpsc.2016.02.016

Krauss R, et al. Recommendations from dietary Guidelines for Healthy American Adults: A statement for health professionals from the Nutrition Committee, American Heart Association. *Circulation.* 1996;94(7):1795–1800.

Lamond AI, Earnshaw WC. Structure and function in the nucleus. *Science.* 1998;280(5363):547–553. doi:10.1126/science.280.5363.547

Lefèvre CT, Bazylinski DA. Ecology, diversity, and evolution of magnetotactic bacteria. *Microbiol Mol Biol Rev.* 2013;77(3):497–526. doi:10.1128/MMBR.00021-13

Lemas DJ, Yee S, Cacho N, Miller D, Cardel M, Gurka M, Janicke D, Shenkman E. Exploring the contribution of maternal antibiotics and breastfeeding to development of the infant microbiome and pediatric obesity. *Semin Fetal Neonatal Med.* 2016;21(6):406–409. doi:10.1016/j.siny.2016.04.013

Li F. Structure, function, and evolution of coronavirus spike proteins. *Annu Rev Virol.* 2016;3(1):237–261. doi:10.1146/annurev-virology-110615-042301

Louten J. Chapter 2: Virus structure and classification. *Essent Hum Virol.* 2016;19–29. doi:10.1016/B978-0-12-800947-5.00002-8

Madhogaria B, Bhowmik P, Kundu A. Correlation between human gut microbiome and diseases, *Infect Med.* 2022;1(3):180–191. doi:10.1016/j.imj.2022.08.004

Magne F, Gotteland M, Gauthier L, Zazueta A, Pesoa S, Navarrete P, Balamurugan R. The firmicutes/bacteroidetes ratio: A relevant marker of gut dysbiosis in obese patients? *Nutrients.* 2020;12(5):1474. doi:10.3390/nu12051474.

Manson JM, Rauch M, Gilmore MS. The commensal microbiology of the gastrointestinal tract. *Adv Exp Med Biol.* 2008;635:15–28. doi:10.1007/978-0-387-09550-9_2

Morrison DJ, Tom Preston T. Formation of short chain fatty acids by the gut microbiota and their impact on human metabolism. *Gut Microbes.* 2016;7(3):189–200. doi:10.1080/19490976.2015.1134082

Murat D, Byrne M, Komeili A. Cell biology of prokaryotic organelles. *Cold Spring Harb Perspect Biol.* 2010;2:a000422.

Myles IA. Fast food fever: Reviewing the impacts of the Western diet on immunity. *Nutr J.* 2014;13:61. doi:10.1186/1475-2891-13-61.

Ogunrinola GA, Oyewale JO, Oshamika OO, Olasehinde GI. The human microbiome and its impacts on health. *Int J Microbiol.* 2020;2020:8045646. Published 2020 June 12. doi:10.1155/2020/8045646

Oh JH, Alexander LM, Pan M, Schueler KL, Keller MP, Attie AD, Walter J, van Pijkeren JP. Dietary fructose and microbiota-derived short-chain fatty acids promote bacteriophage production in the gut symbiont Lactobacillus reuteri. *Cell Host Microbe.* 2019;25(2):273–284.e6. doi:10.1016/j.chom.2018.11.016

Opron K, Burton ZF. Ribosome structure, function, and early evolution. *Int J Mol Sci.* 2019; 20:40. doi:10.3390/ijms20010040

Pace NR. A molecular view of microbial diversity and the biosphere. *Science.* 1997; 276(5313): 734–740. doi:10.1126/science.276.5313.734

Pan XD, Chen FQ, Wu TX, Tang HG, Zhao ZY. Prebiotic oligosaccharides change the concentrations of short-chain fatty acids and the microbial population of mouse bowel. *J Zhejiang Univ Sci B.* 2009;10(4):258–263. doi:10.1631/jzus.B0820261

Pascal M, Perez-Gordo M, Caballero T, Escribese MM, Lopez Longo MN, Luengo O, Manso L, Matheu V, Seoane E, Zamorano M, Labrador M, Mayorga C. Microbiome and allergic diseases. *Front Immunol.* 2018;9:1584. doi:10.3389/fimmu.2018.01584

Pederson T. The nucleus introduced. *Cold Spring Harb Perspect Biol.* 2011;3(5):a000521. doi:10.1101/cshperspect.a000521

Portincasa P, Bonfrate L, Vacca M, De Angelis M, Farella I, Lanza E, Khalil M, Wang DQ, Sperandio M, Di Ciaula A. Gut microbiota and short chain fatty acids: Implications in glucose homeostasis. *Int J Mol Sci.* 2022;23(3):1105. doi:10.3390/ijms23031105

Qi L. Fried foods, gut microbiota, and glucose metabolism. *Diabetes Care.* 2021;44(9):1907–1909. doi:10.2337/dci21-0033

Rinninella E, Raoul P, Cintoni M, Franceschi F, Miggiano GAD, Gasbarrini A, Mele MC. What is the healthy gut microbiota composition? A changing ecosystem across age, environment, diet, and diseases. *Microorganisms.* 2019;7(1):14. doi:10.3390/microorganisms7010014

Santacroce L, Charitos IA, Ballini A, Inchingolo F, Luperto P, De Nitto E, Topi S. The human respiratory system and its microbiome at a glimpse. *Biology.* 2020;9:318. doi:10.3390/biology9100318

Sanvictores T, Davis DD. Histology, rough endoplasmic reticulum. [Updated 2023 Aug 8]. In *StatPearls.* Treasure Island, FL: StatPearls Publishing; 2024. www.ncbi.nlm.nih.gov/books/NBK563126/

Sender R, Fuchs S, Milo R. Are we really vastly outnumbered? Revisiting the ratio of bacterial to host cells in humans. *Cell.* 2016;164(3):337–340. doi:10.1016/j.cell.2016.01.013

Silva YP, Bernardi A, Frozza RL. The role of short-chain fatty acids from gut microbiota in gut-brain communication. *Front Endocrinol.* 2020;11.

Singh RK, Chang HW, Yan D, Lee KM, Ucmak D, Wong K, Abrouk M, Farahnik B, Nakamura M, Zhu TH, Bhutani T, Liao W. Influence of diet on the gut microbiome and implications for human health. *J Transl Med.* 2017;15(1):73. doi:10.1186/s12967-017-1175-y

Sokolowska M, Frei R, Lunjani N, Akdis CA, O'Mahony L. Microbiome and asthma. *Asthma Res Pract.* 2018;4:1. doi:10.1186/s40733-017-0037-y

Su C, Lei L, Duan Y, Zhang KQ, Yang J. Culture-independent methods for studying environmental microorganisms: Methods, application, and perspective. *Appl. Microbiol. Biotechnol.* 2012;93(3):993–1003. doi:10.1007/s00253-011-3800-7

Tan J, McKenzie C, Potamitis M, Thorburn AN, et al. Chapter 3: The role of short-chain fatty acids in health and disease. In Alt FW, editor. *Advances in Immunology* (Volume 121). Academic Press; 2014:91–119. doi:10.1016/B978-0-12-800100-4.00003-9.

Townsend GE, Han W, Schwalm ND, Raghavan V, Barry NA, Goodman AL, Groisman EA. Dietary sugar silences a colonization factor in a mammalian gut symbiont. *Proc Nat Acad Sci.* 2019;116(1):233–238. doi:10.1073/pnas.1813780115

Ursell LK, Metcalf JL, Parfrey LW, Knight R. Defining the human microbiome. *Nut Rev.* 2012;70(Suppl 1):S38. doi:10.1111/j.1753-4887.2012.00493.x

Weinstock GM. Genomic approaches to studying the human microbiota. *Nature.* 2012;489(7415):250–256. doi:10.1038/nature11553

Wheelis M, Kandler O, Woese CR. On the nature of global classification. *Proc. Nati. Acad. Sci. USA.* 1992;89:2930–2934.

Wright RG, Bottino PJ. Mitochondrial DNA. *Sci Teach.* 1986;53(4):27–31. www.jstor.org/stable/24140078 (Accessed 1 September 2023).

Young V. The role of the microbiome in human health and disease: An Introduction for clinicians. *BMJ.* 2017;356:j831.

Zhou X, Liao WJ, Liao JM, Liao P, Lu H. Ribosomal proteins: Functions beyond the ribosome. *J Mol Cell Biol.* 2015;7(2):92–104. doi:10.1093/jmcb/mjv014

Zinöcker MK, Lindseth IA. The western diet – microbiome-host interaction and its role in metabolic disease. *Nutrients.* 2018;10(3):365. doi:10.3390/nu10030365

CHAPTER 7

On the Importance of Being Physically Active

7.0 Introduction

At every stage of life, regular physical activity is beneficial. Physical activity, and especially exercise, by design, leads to positive health outcomes. In fact, as noted by Fletcher and colleagues (2018), physical inactivity is one of the most important modifiable risk factors to support cardiovascular health. The benefits of physical activity and planned, purposeful exercise at specific magnitudes of intensity are not only associated with cardiovascular disease prevention, but the benefits of being physically active support positive states of social, emotional, and physical health across all age groups (Hargreaves, 2021). There is a plethora of research on the benefits of being physically active daily, and the overwhelming evidence that your health (not merely the absence of disease or infirmity) and the health of the planet benefits from pursuing or maintaining levels of physical fitness throughout the life cycle (Mahmood et al., 2014; Tsao and Vasan, 2015). Moreover, there is a teleological argument – from the Greek word *telos* (end, goal, purpose) and *logos* (reason, explanation) – that we should strive to support systems that promote physical activity in the form of exercise in our daily lives. As a society, we should promote and support opportunities for people to be physically active daily, if not for us, then for all the elements of the planet in the future.

7.1 Defining Physical Activity and Exercise

Let's begin by defining physical activity. Physical activity (PA), as formerly defined by Caspersen et al. (1985), is any bodily movement that is produced by skeletal muscles and therefore requires energy expenditure by the individual. In establishing this definition, Caspersen and coworkers, described physical activity based on energy expenditure measured in kilocalories (a measure of heat units). They used a simple categorization of physical activity that ranged from activities while sleeping through to activities while working and also activities while at leisure. However, while they included a simple formula to quantify the energy expended during such activities, given here as:

DOI: 10.4324/9781003474777-7

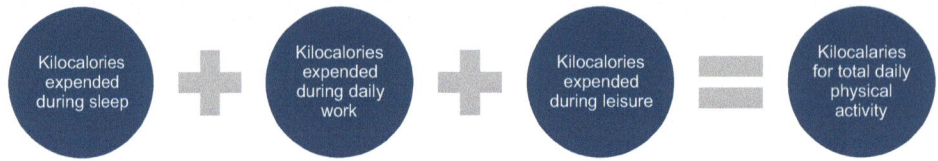

Figure 7.1 A formula to quantify energy expended.

the breakdown of activities is extremely gross and does not provide sufficient measures of sensitivity (ability to discriminate differences) or specificity (ability to show precision or accuracy).

To advance the definition of physical activity that would be more inclusive of an individual's lived experience, Piggin (2020) proposed that physical activity be described from a holistic perspective as that which ***involves people moving, acting, and performing within culturally specific spaces and contexts and influenced by a unique array of interests, emotions, ideas, instructions, and relationships.***

This definition is certainly more holistic, more health centric, and less focused on merely the physicality of movement. In the Piggin definition, the author considers movement from multiple perspectives that intentionally extends beyond the biomedical and epidemiological foundations of movement and thus includes considerations for the politics of movement, the emotion and creativity of movement, the cognition, motivation, and planning of movement, and especially the sociocultural aspects of movement. Equally important is what this new definition implicitly avoids, and that is the overmedicalization of movement or the reporting of movement to be purposeful as a function of some arbitrary, externally measured worth. In this regard, however, the author has not eliminated the importance of movement to the epidemiological evidence of physical health and disease-prevention outcomes gained through involvement in regular physical activity. However, by applying a more holistic lens, that is a lens which considers that physical activity describes a gestalt which is bigger than the sum of its parts, Piggin proposes a definition that fits well with the larger principles of health, which is to consider movement as an essential partner for all of the principles of health in the broadest perspective.

Comparing and contrasting the term *physical activity* with the term *exercise* demonstrates the profound differences which exist between these two pursuits. While physical activity is ***any*** body movement, Caspersen et al. (1985) defined exercise as a specific type of physical movement – activity that is planned and structured with the explicit purpose of improving physical fitness and gaining health benefits. The general conjecture of equating exercise to physical fitness and disease prevention is easily measured through many epidemiological applications but restricted predominantly to the physical dimensions of health. The inference of this approach is that if we can improve an individual's physical fitness, which we can measure through both direct laboratory tests and indirect field tests, then we can reduce the risk factors that are attributed to specific types of illness and disabilities and thereby improve an individual's health status.

Limited as it may seem, adopting a regimen of regular physical exercise has been shown to have tremendous benefits beyond the dimensions of physical health. Pursuing exercise which is planned and purposeful extends mental health benefits through establishing routines and expressing work outputs at a level that can invoke deep meditative states and connect to one's inner self. Likewise, planned and purposeful activities, which can be done in groups through team-based activities or which, when pursued individually, can establish an identity to a cohort of like-minded individuals. This, in turn, can catalyze the formation of social groups that continue to provide social support well beyond the exercise environment.

Exercise and physical activity are two essential elements that support the development of one's health. Both exercise and physical activity describe constructs which, although related, are also independent and can be studied separately. We could consider physical activity as the foundation, whereas exercise describes an application of physical activity that may be intentional, that may be planned, and that may be purposefully associated with a defined outcome. Taken in this way, both physical activity and exercise will have characteristics that are described uniquely, but both exercise and physical activity will contribute to our health in its holism.

7.2 On the Relationship Between Physical Activity and Mental Health

Although many epidemiological studies describe the health benefits of involvement in regular physical activity as pertaining to the reduction in chronic disease risk factors and outcomes, research evidence supports that pursuits to improve one's physical fitness lead to measurable psychological benefits that are directly attributed to being physically active regularly (Overdorf et al., 2016). In a study published by Chekroud et al. (2018), the researchers showed that between 2011 and 2015, for a sample of more than 1.2 million U.S. participants, individuals who indicated that they participated in regular exercise had just under one and a half fewer days of poor mental health in the past month compared to individuals who did not exercise. This rate of positive mental health days translates to a 43.2% decrease in poor-mental-health days among the exercisers. This trend in beneficial effect was observed across all exercise types that were measured within the sample and translates to a range of 11.8% to 22.3% reduction in poor health days for all activity participation. Interestingly, the activities that showed the greatest reduction were team sports, cycling, and gym/aerobic activities. However, the authors also noted that more exercise was not necessarily better and that exercise type, duration, and how often an individual engaged in physical activity were fundamental to establishing volumetric clinical prescription targets when striving to reduce mental health burden.

Several studies have shown a relationship between subjective assessment of mood states – depression and anxiety – following regular participation in a regimen of planned physical activities (Graham et al., 2019; Zschucke et al., 2013). The findings of Chekroud and coworkers are consistent with those of Bowe et al. (2018) for a sample of more than 7,500 participants from Ireland. In their study, the researchers showed that individuals who self-classified as non-exercisers were three times less likely to report positive mental health states and three times more likely to report negative mental health.

Aside from the inherent importance of depression and anxiety as conditions with significant health and societal impacts, depression has been implicated in the earlier onset of mild cognitive impairment (MCI), dementia, and Alzheimer's disease (AD). Reduction or loss of cognitive functioning in older adults is an increasingly problematic reality with serious consequences for the person, family, and society. Research by Gomez-Pinilla and Hillman (2013) reported that involvement in planned physical activities has positive effects on the maintenance of cognitive functions across the lifespan. Moreover, in aging individuals, regular participation in exercise programs can inhibit the loss of brain tissue, which is a natural function of the aging process, and, in so doing, can maintain and even enhance the patterns of functionality of those regions of the brain that are involved in cognition. Importantly, the researchers alluded to the importance of the volumetric load of activity, stating that individuals who were more active and subsequently had higher relative levels of physical fitness had a greater likelihood to allocate attentional resources to tasks and process information quicker. Demonstrating such utility is surely an evolutionary trait one could consider inherent to survival mechanisms. The research of Gomez-Pinilla and Hillman not only describes correlative and observational findings of previous research but also reports on benchtop studies that support distinct physical adaptations in brain physiology that result from involvement in planned and purposeful activities across the lifespan.

7.3 Aging, Physical Activity, and Activities of Daily Living

At this point, a consideration of activities of daily living (ADL) and especially a comment on instrumental activities of daily living is important to our discussion on why maintaining regular physical activity is essential for positive states of health. The ADL are defined as the basic personal tasks that individuals perform each day (Wang et al., 2020; LaPlante, 2010). These activities are often performed independently but may be influenced negatively by the process of aging and the effects of disability. Activities of daily living include bathing, using the toilet, moving in and out of bed, having control of urination and defecation, and being able to feed oneself (LaPlante, 2010). These are essential activities that decline with age and are indicators of increasing morbidity (Diehr et al., 2013). As research into the nomenclature of activities of daily living expanded, the original ADL categorization was subdivided into eight distinct domains of functionality by Lawton and Brody (1969) and referred to as Instrumental Activities of Daily Living (IADL). As noted by Carmona-Torres et al. (2019), IADLs refer to daily operational activities that are more complex and often require higher levels of cognition and autonomy, like using the telephone, purchasing groceries, and preparing meals, as well as performing those duties associated with housekeeping and doing the laundry, using transportation, taking regular medications, and managing personal finances (LaPlante, 2010).

Both the health- and skill-related outcomes from daily involvement in physical activity pursuits lead to improvements in agility and balance, greater aerobic and anaerobic capacity, enhanced proportional body composition, cardiorespiratory endurance, flexibility, muscular endurance and muscular strength, a greater capacity to cope with stress, and realizing the joie de vivre (Hurtig-Wennlöf et al., 2007).

The normal chores that younger persons take for granted and assume have minimal physical requirements, such as vacuuming, raking leaves, shoveling snow, or performing active transport as in walking or cycling to school or work, or even engaging in active recreation like walking a pet, jogging, strolling, or even spoiling a good walk by playing golf, can be insurmountable for aging individuals.

7.4 Cancers, Insulin, and Type 2 Diabetes

Involvement in daily physical activity can reduce the risk factors related to cancer.

Working to improve an individual's risk for chronic disease begins by establishing those factors that can be modified. Evidence from epidemiological research at the population level supports the contention that improving an individual's physical fitness through regular participation in moderate to vigorous aerobic physical activity (MVPA) and muscle-strengthening activity (MSA) can not only restore physical health status, as we see in rehabilitation settings, but can also prevent the progression of risk factors known to be precursors to chronic disease (Bennie et al., 2019).

Moore and coworkers (2016) noted that leisure-time physical activity at a moderate to high level was associated with the reduction in risk factors for as many as 13 different types of cancers which included colon, breast, esophageal, liver, lung, rectal, gastric, bladder, and kidney cancers, to name a few. Most important, the risk factor reductions for these cancers did not show a preferential outcome as a function of body mass, which means that regardless of body weight, the risk factor benefit between leisure-time physical activity and cancer was the same, making these findings much more relevant to the general population. Conversely, it is important to note that in the work by Moore et al., leisure-time physical activity was associated with higher risk factors for malignant melanoma and prostate cancer. A similar review study of cancer risk factor reduction associated with exercise by Farris and coworkers (2015) showed that involvement in regularly scheduled leisure-time physical activity had a protective association with pancreatic cancer, based on an estimated 95% confidence interval for relative risk estimates being below 1.00. In their review of some 26 eligible studies, Farris reported that there was an 11% risk reduction in developing pancreatic cancer when the individual was involved in regular leisure-time physical activity. These findings are important because they provide additional evidence that exercise has a positive protective association with pancreatic cancer, which Bao and Michaud (2008) were unable to show from their earlier work.

The link between pancreatic cancer and physical activity is worth exploring further, and not only because it is among the most prevalent cancer-based causes of death for adults or because individuals generally do not recognize the symptoms until late in the disease progression when the metastasis is rapid, meaning that it spreads quickly and has often been reported to lead to death within one year of diagnosis (Bao and Michaud, 2008). But more importantly, pancreatic cancer is a disease that is associated with type 2 diabetes, and type 2 diabetes is a disease that exercise can affect directly in a positive way. Type 2 diabetes is a progressive disease that results from an individual's inability to effectively use the hormone insulin to move blood sugar (glucose) into cells, where it is either stored or used directly to produce energy through either the anaerobic metabolism of glycolysis or the aerobic metabolism of the Krebs Cycle.

Blood glucose is a sugar that we derive from our consumption of carbohydrates. When we eat a meal, the gastrointestinal degradation of the foodstuff leads to an increase in the concentration of blood glucose. The post-meal increase in the concentration of blood glucose (hyperglycemia) stimulates the pancreas to release the hormone insulin. Insulin is responsible for moving the glucose molecule from normal blood flow either into the liver, where the glucose is stored as glycogen for later use in energy production, or directly into muscle tissue, where the glucose molecule is used in intermediary metabolic processes, both anaerobically and aerobically, to produce energy in the form of adenosine triphosphate (ATP).

However, when an individual becomes insulin resistant, that is, their cells are resistant to the effects of insulin and the normal uptake of blood glucose by the cells is inhibited, the efficiency of glucose mobilization from blood to tissue is reduced. The concomitant effect of insulin resistance is an inability to use glucose as a fuel in normal cellular metabolism.

Insulin sensitivity is the opposite of insulin resistance. Insulin sensitivity is the responsivity of the cells to enable glucose uptake from blood to tissue in the presence of insulin. As Ross (2003) indicated, exercise, even at a moderate level, can increase the body's ability to overcome insulin resistance and improve the insulin sensitivity response. Participating in regular physical activity reduces the risk factors associated with the progression of type 2 diabetes by enhancing the sensitivity of cells to insulin and maintaining appropriate levels of blood glucose.

Type 2 diabetes represents one of the lifestyle diseases. That is, type 2 diabetes represents one of the chronic diseases that results from our lifestyle behaviors and is therefore preventable. For many of us living in countries where we have access to fresh water, shelter, and safe environments, our lifestyle is one of the most important contributors to the progression of diseases that can directly influence our ability to achieve a healthy state. Preventable chronic diseases include but are not limited to cardiovascular disease (including stroke as well as coronary heart disease), type 2 diabetes, cancers, and lung diseases. Liver cirrhosis from abuse of alcohol, obesity associated with sedentary behaviors, osteoporosis, and gastrointestinal cancers from the overconsumption of nitrosamines – the chemicals used to cure meats and fish – are also considered among the preventable chronic diseases. While exercise – physical activity that is planned and purposeful – is not a panacea for preventable chronic diseases, it has tremendous evidence-based positive influences on controlling the risk factors for such lifestyle-related diseases. Risk factors for preventable chronic diseases are especially influenced by the frequency, intensity, and duration of our exercise regimens as shown through a comprehensive review of several studies by Swain and Franklin (2006).

As adults, we need to be physically active, at a moderate to vigorous intensity, for at least 30 minutes each day. While we have heard this mantra many times, we also need to consider that the exercise we plan is not only limited to simple movements that engage our cardio (heart) and respiratory (lungs) systems as we move. As adults who are aging at a rate beyond that which we allow ourselves to believe, we need to maintain (and, for many of us, enhance) our current levels of strength and flexibility. Being able to walk to the store to purchase healthy foods is important, but being able to bend over to tie our shoelaces and carry our purchases back home is as essential to reducing the risk factors that lead to negative health outcomes. From an exercise perspective, our daily – yes, DAILY – exercise regimen must consider three simple principles in order to capture the overall benefits of physical activity for reducing preventable chronic disease risk factors. Our exercise regimen must include breathing, bending, and overcoming resistance. The principle of breathing is the easiest to consider, as it is the core of most exercise programs. In Canada, for several years, PARTICIPACTION promoted the slogan "Walk a block a day" to encourage individuals to get out and move at least the distance of an urban city block every day. Evidence associated with participation in regular exercise programs that include even low- to moderate-intensity activities like walking is overwhelmingly convincing (Warburton et al., 2006; Manson et al., 2002; Morris and Hardman, 1997). As noted, when individuals maintain a program of regular moderate-intensity activity, they gain benefits across the spectrum of health. Not only does the individual reduce their risk of death from cardiovascular-related diseases, but as Morris and Hardman indicated, they realize the psychological and social benefits from getting out into the environment and interacting with like-minded individuals.

Yet as we begin to plan our exercise behaviors, we need to consider the research by Hamilton and coworkers (2008), which showed that just getting up off the couch is as important as jumping into action with our daily exercise regimen. In their review, the researchers showed that while being physically active was essential to reducing risk factors associated with the preventable chronic diseases, avoiding sedentary behaviors was independently associated with controlling similar risk factors. Hamilton et al. reported evidence that by remaining sedentary, we are not only missing the benefits of physical activity for enhancing metabolic systems that reduce risk factors, but we may also be enhancing the metabolic and genetic mechanisms that predispose us to preventable chronic diseases. The summary conclusion by Hamilton and coworkers was simple – "stand more and sit less."

7.5 Cardiovascular Disease Within the Forgotten Cohort – Aka Women

Until the COVID-19 pandemic in 2020, North Americans rarely worried about infectious diseases as the major cause of death in society. Rather, our primary focus in healthcare and especially in achieving positive states of health was more on those behaviors which could be considered as fundamental to lifestyle. Recapping what we know, being physically active can help to control the risk of cardiovascular disease as well as type 2 diabetes by improving glucose metabolism and reducing body fat storage while using fat as a fuel in energy production. Planned physical activity, as in regular exercise, can help to regulate blood pressure and reduce the risk factors associated with hypertension. Maintaining a regular regimen of moderate- to vigorous-intensity exercise for at least 30 minutes each day will prevent the progression of cardiovascular disease.

As noted by the World Health Organization (2024) cardiovascular disease, more specifically coronary or ischemic heart disease, is the leading non-communicable cause of death worldwide. Coronary heart disease is described as cardiovascular disease in which there is an inability to deliver oxygenated blood to the myocardium, the heart muscle. Similarly, the atherosclerotic plaque that clogs the coronary vessels that supply oxygen to the heart also clogs the peripheral vasculature that supplies oxygenated blood to the tissues throughout the body.

Both coronary vascular (artery) disease and peripheral vascular disease are caused by narrowing of the arteries because of blockage due to the progressive condition of atherosclerotic plaque. In Canada, where cardiovascular disease is the second leading cause of death after cancer (CCDSS, 2018), approximately 8% of the adult population over the age of 20 have been diagnosed with the disease. Representing the disease as a proportion of the population, we can say that some 1 in 12 Canadians is affected by the progressive characteristics of atherosclerosis, leading to cardiovascular disease. Conditions such as obesity, diabetes, and hypertension, the condition that is characterized as having blood pressure readings above the normal readings of 120 over 80 (which means 120 mmHg systolic pressure and 80 mmHg diastolic pressure), are known contributing factors to cardiovascular disease, and as such, they increase the prevalence of cardiovascular disease both nationally and globally.

The impact of cardiovascular disease on death rate and loss of quality-of-life years remaining is so profound that if we were to eliminate all forms of cardiovascular disease, life expectancy would rise measurably. In fact, in a study by Li et al. (2018), the researchers noted that in the United States, if 50-year-olds followed a low-risk lifestyle that included never smoking, maintaining a body mass index of 18.5 to 24.9 kg/m^2, increasing their physical activity levels to be at the moderate to vigorous level for more than 30 minutes per day, and moderating their alcohol intake while improving their diet, they could increase their life expectancy by 14 years for females and 12.2 years for males.

As Woodward (2019) reported, coronary heart disease (CHD) is the most common cause of death among women in developed countries. Comparatively, in the developing countries, where life struggles and environmental risk factors are clearly different than those of the developed countries, coronary heart disease ranks fifth among most common causes of death amongst women. Organization of CHD related data comparing death rates among males and females shows us that even though most may believe the disease to be the likely killer of middle-aged males, proportional death rates of females are certainly on par with those reported for males. In 2017, Keteepe-Arachi and Sharma reported that some 2.8 million women in the UK were diagnosed with cardiovascular disease (CVD), and although this was an accurate rate for the women who sought healthcare, the researchers suggested that the overall diagnosis of CVD among females was under reported; hence, the actual death rate due to CVD would also be considered underreported. Failing to recognize the prevalence of CVD among women is a forerunner to underdiagnosis, which can, in turn, lead to a lack of attention to the early warning signs and symptoms of CVD in the female cohort.

For example, Garcia et al. (2016) reported that female patients, in comparison to male counterparts with similar disease risk factors, were less likely to receive the essential CVD prevention regimens that males would be provided, such as prescriptions for lipid-lowering pharmaceuticals, including a daily low-dose acetylsalicylic acid (ASA) or suggested changes in lifestyle behaviors. Likewise, Garcia noted that even when women were identified to have progressive CVD, the treatment they received was less aggressive compared to that of males with similar conditions. These differences in disease approaches that include prevention, diagnosis, treatment, and evaluation are the causal contributors to an observable sex-based mortality gap.

In their comprehensive review of cardiovascular disease in women, Garcia and coworkers describe both the traditional and non-traditional risk factors for CVD among women. For example, the traditional risk factors (those that we have seen in studies of male cohorts with suspected atherosclerotic vascular disease) include diabetes mellitus, hypertension, dyslipidemia, smoking, obesity, and physical inactivity. However, they also provided a list of non-traditional and emerging risk factors for CVD among women including preterm delivery, hypertensive pregnancy disorders, gestational diabetes mellitus, breast cancer treatments, autoimmune diseases, and depression.

Reflective of the earlier work by Mosca (2007), there continues to be investigative work to support the development of sex-specific guidelines that can be used to build algorithms that will not only identify women at risk for CVD but provide guidelines for disease progression. Certainly, most of us believe we have reached a point at which disparities in cardiovascular care because of racial, ethnic, and sex differences is no long acceptable in society in general and in healthcare specifically. However, research by Balla et al. (2020) would suggest that those of us that think this way must be ideologically out of touch with reality. Disparities in prevention, diagnosis, treatment, and evaluation continue to be biased along racial, ethnic, and sex categories. That is, research continues to show that CVD risk factors differ between males and females, with women only demonstrating gestational diabetes and pre-eclampsia, but then there are also risk factors associated with psychosocial variables such as depression and anxiety, provision of childcare, and responsibilities as a homemaker, all of which are subdivided according to race and ethnicity.

Recognizing the limitations resulting from implicit bias and acting on the recognition of implicit bias may be a first step in dealing with the observable and measurable sex-based mortality gap.

7.6 Societal Implications of Physical Inactivity

Poor health costs lots of money, but not just from direct medical costs; you really can't forget about the indirect costs. While Mozaffarian et al. (2015) showed that the cost of heart disease in the U.S. in 2011 was approximately $215.6 billion, this did not include costs associated with hypertension ($46.4 billion), stroke ($33.6 billion), and the catch-all category of other cardiovascular diseases ($24.6 billion). The direct costs are typically reported as physician and nursing services, in-hospital care charges, nursing home services, medications, and various home healthcare needs. In addition, there are the indirect costs associated with cardiovascular disease such as loss of productivity due to illness, absenteeism/replacement workers, health insurance increases, family hardship, and decreased-quality-of-life years remaining.

Global trends in physical inactivity indicate that world-wide, more than 60% of adults do not engage in sufficient levels of physical activity which are beneficial to their health. Moreover, physical inactivity is more prevalent among women, older adults, individuals from low socioeconomic groups, and the disabled. Physical activity also decreases with age during adolescence, and this decline continues throughout the adult years. In many countries, developed and developing, less than one-third of young people are sufficiently active to benefit their present and future health, and most often, the research evidence finds that female adolescents are less active than male adolescents.

In Canada, as you might expect, the data indicate that males report more activity than females and that younger persons report more activity involvement than older adults. In Canada, Janssen (2012) and Colley et al. (2011) considered that some 85% of Canadian adults do not meet Canada's physical activity guidelines of 150 minutes per week of moderate to vigorous physical activity. Additionally, when reviewing the costs of physical inactivity, Janssen estimated that being physically inactive led to a value of $6.8 billion (CDN) and represented 3.7% of total healthcare costs.

> **So why do such constraints on being physically active exist within society?**

For some, it is the issue of health literacy and the lack of awareness about the overall health benefits of maintaining a level of physical activity. Given Janssen's research, only 15% of the Canadian population accept that positive health outcomes can be gained from regular involvement in activities that are planned and purposeful despite that statements of such benefits are evidenced based. We know that being physically active daily has positive health benefits, and research also supports that there are both intrinsic and extrinsic motivators for adopting a lifestyle that includes a daily regimen of physical activity (Galan-Lopez et al., 2022). Yet that is not enough to convince the population that physical activity is a determinant of health. Awareness is one consideration, but the importance of political will and thus political commitment through explicit support, as in generating opportunities for active transport, helping individuals to participate, creating policies to remove barriers to involvement, and improving educational messaging across the lifespan, are essential to improving participation rates (GAPA, 2011). Governments must become the drivers of change by enhancing the accessibility and availability of activity facilities for the entire public and not merely to those who can afford to pay for access. Consider, for example, accessibility to public skating within communities versus access to paid recreational leagues such as ringette and ice hockey. The economic costs associated with participation in physical activity is one of the strongest barriers to engaging in certain types of physical activity. Yet the importance of some of the activities is also questionable when we consider the economic burden of participation, the injury risks associated with participation, the environmental effects of participation, and the attitudes about the importance that society places on participating in certain activities.

As in all aspects of nature, there exists a light side and a dark side. Sport and physical activity are not differently influenced by this counterpoise. The influence of financial prosperity that can be attributed directly to success in sport has led to many of the events on the dark side of sport, while the development of physical, mental, and social health through positive team building, increased self-esteem, and connectivity across the social fabric of societies represents some of the positive attributes of the light side. As health promoters, educators, practitioners, and policymakers, we are challenged to navigate the regions of the counterpoise between the light and dark sides of physical activity to enable the greatest involvement of society in sport, physical activity, and recreation. Our responsibility is to continue working toward establishing positive attitudes toward physical activity involvement so that we can increase participation and thereby reap greater benefits as a civilization.

7.7 Forest Bathing and Non-Traditional Physical Activities

> *We cannot expect to change activity rates if we do not change our attitudes about the types of activities in which we participate and the overall importance of physical activity in our lives.*

As we consider the benefits of exercise on enhancing our health, let's consider the psychological impact of place of activity on health outcomes. The term *forest bathing*, which in Japan is known as *shinrin-yoku*, was described by Mao et al. (2012) and Song et al. (2019) and Wen et al. (2019) as having benefits that extend beyond the physical to psychosocial and even economic impacts for enhancement of green spaces versus construction of housing (Tyrväinen, 2001) or the perceived emotional and intellectual values (Peckham et al., 2013). Exercising in environments that are free of pollution (air and noise) and which convey a feeling of calm serenity and security has been shown to increase positive mental health while reducing reports of negative psychological outcomes. For example, Song and coworkers (2019) reported that when comparing the outcomes of walking through forests versus walking through urban areas, participants reported improved positive mood states based on measures of perceived vigor and reductions in their negative mood states based on scores for perceived states of depression-dejection tension-anxiety, anger-hostility, fatigue, and confusion.

As we gain a greater understanding of health as being not merely the absence of disease or infirmity, we can become promoters of health and contribute positively to society. We can promote health and wellness by providing evidence to support claims that exercise and physical activity have direct and indirect cost benefits as well as social, emotional, and physical benefits for the health of individuals. Likewise, we can demonstrate through our support and behavior that involvement in regular exercise can prevent illness and disability and help to restore health through rehabilitation.

7.7.1 Discussion Questions

1   What is the influence of participation in regular physical activity on mental health and mood states? What kinds of programs are most likely to provide the greatest return on our health?
2   How might we promote physical activity participation across the lifespan, across cultures, and especially among individuals within marginalized cohorts?

References

Balla S, Gomez SE, Rodriguez F. Disparities in cardiovascular care and outcomes for women from racial/ethnic minority backgrounds. *Curr Treat Options Cardiovasc Med.* 2020;22(12):75. doi:10.1007/s11936-020-00869-z

Bao Y, Michaud DS. Physical activity and pancreatic cancer risk: A systematic review. *Cancer Epidemiol Biomarkers Prev.* 2008;17(10):2671–2682. doi:10.1158/1055-9965.EPI-08-0488

Bennie JA, De Cocker K, Teychenne MJ, et al. The epidemiology of aerobic physical activity and muscle-strengthening activity guideline adherence among 383,928 U.S. adults. *Int J Behav Nutr Phys Act.* 2019;16:34. doi:10.1186/s12966-019-0797-2

Bowe AK, Owens M, Codd MB, Lawlor BA, Glynn RW. Physical activity and mental health in an Irish population. *Ir J Med Sci.* 2019;188(2):625–631. doi:10.1007/s11845-018-1863-5

Carmona-Torres JM, Rodríguez-Borrego MA, Laredo-Aguilera JA, López-Soto PJ, Santacruz-Salas E, Cobo-Cuenca AI. Disability for basic and instrumental activities of daily living in older individuals. *PLoS One.* 2019;14(7):e0220157. doi:10.1371/journal.pone.0220157

Caspersen CJ, Powell KE, Christenson GM. Physical activity, exercise, and physical fitness: Definitions and distinctions for health-related research. *Pub Health Rep.* 1985;100(2):126–131.

CCDSS Report on Cardiovascular Disease in Canada. WHO statement on CVD as cause of Death (see notes in File Chapter 7). 2018. www.who.int/news-room/fact-sheets/detail/the-top-10-causes-of-death (accessed 1 February 2021).

Chekroud SR, Gueorguieva R, Zheutlin AB, et al. Association between physical exercise and mental health in 1·2 million individuals in the USA between 2011 and 2015: A cross-sectional study. *Lancet Psychiat.* 2018;5(9):739–746. doi:10.1016/S2215-0366(18)30227-X

Colley RC, Garriguet D, Janssen I, Craig CL, Clarke J, Tremblay MS. Physical activity of Canadian adults: Accelerometer results from the 2007 to 2009 Canadian Health Measures Survey. *Health Rep.* 2011;22(1):7–14.

Diehr PH, Thielke SM, Newman AB, Hirsch C, Tracy R. Decline in health for older adults: Five-year change in 13 key measures of standardized health. *J Gerontol A Biol Sci Med Sci.* 2013;68(9):1059–1067. doi:10.1093/gerona/glt038

Eisenmann JC. Physical activity and cardiovascular disease risk factors in children and adolescents: An overview. *Can J Cardiol.* 2004;20(3):295–301.

Ekkekakis P, Swinton P, Tiller NB. Extraordinary claims in the literature on high-intensity interval training (HIIT): I. Bonafide scientific revolution or a looming crisis of replication and credibility? *Sports Med.* 2023;53(10):1865–1890. doi:10.1007/s40279-023-01880-7

Farris MS, Mosli MH, McFadden AA, Friedenreich CM, Brenner DR. The association between leisure time physical activity and pancreatic cancer risk in adults: A systematic review and meta-analysis. *Cancer Epidemiol Biomarkers Prev.* 2015;24(10):1462–1473. doi:10.1158/1055-9965.EPI-15-0301

Fletcher GF, Landolfo C, Niebauer J, et al. Promoting physical activity and exercise. *J Am Coll Cardiol.* 2018;72(23):3053–3070.

Galan-Lopez P, Lopez-Cobo I, García-Lázaro I, Ries F. Associations between motives for physical exercise, body composition and cardiorespiratory fitness: A cross-sectional study. *Int J Environ Res Public Health.* 2022;19(21):14128. doi:10.3390/ijerp92114128

Garcia M, Mulvagh SL, Merz CN, Buring JE, Manson JE. Cardiovascular disease in women: Clinical perspectives. *Circ Res.* 2016;118(8):1273–1293. doi:10.1161/CIRCRESAHA.116.307547

Global Advocacy for Physical Activity (GAPA) the Advocacy Council of the International Society for Physical Activity and Health (ISPAH). NCD prevention: Investments that work for physical activity. February 2011. www.globalpa.org.uk/investmentsthatwork

Gomez-Pinilla F, Hillman C. The influence of exercise on cognitive abilities. *Compr Physiol.* 2013;3(1):403–428. doi:10.1002/cphy.c110063

Graham S, Depp C, Lee EE, et al. Artificial intelligence for mental health and mental illnesses: An overview. *Curr Psychiat Rep.* 2019;21(11):116. doi:10.1007/s11920-019-1094-0

Hamilton MT, Healy GN, Dunstan DW, Zderic TW, Owen N. Too little exercise and too much sitting: Inactivity physiology and the need for new recommendations on sedentary behavior. *Curr Cardiovasc Risk Rep.* 2008;2(4):292–298. doi:10.1007/s12170-008-0054-8

Hargreaves M. Exercise and health: Historical perspectives and new insights. *J Appl Physiol.* 2021;131(2):575–588.

Hurtig-Wennlöf A, Ruiz JR, Harro M, Sjöström M. Cardiorespiratory fitness relates more strongly than physical activity to cardiovascular disease risk factors in healthy children and adolescents: The European Youth Heart Study. *Eur J Cardiovasc Prev Rehabil.* 2007;14(4):575–581. doi:10.1097/HJR.0b013e32808c67e3

Janssen I. Health care costs of physical inactivity in Canadian adults. *Appl Physiol Nutr Metab.* 2012;37(4):803–806. https://doi.org/10.1139/h2012-061

Keteepe-Arachi T, Sharma S. Cardiovascular disease in women: Understanding symptoms and risk factors. *Eur Cardiol.* 2017;12(1):10–13. doi:10.15420/ecr.2016:32:1

LaPlante MP. The classic measure of disability in activities of daily living is biased by age but an expanded IADL/ADL measure is not. *J Gerontol B Psychol Sci Soc Sci.* 2010;65(6):720–732. doi:10.1093/geronb/gbp129

Lawton MP, Brody EM. Assessment of older people: Self-maintaining and instrumental activities of daily living. *Gerontologist.* 1969;9:179–186.

Li Y, Pan A, Wang DD, et al. Impact of healthy lifestyle factors on life expectancies in the US population. *Circulation.* 2018;138(4):345–355.

Mahmood SS, Levy D, Vasan RS, Wang TJ. The Framingham Heart Study and the epidemiology of cardiovascular disease: A historical perspective. *Lancet.* 2014;383(9921):999–1008. doi:10.1016/S0140-6736(13)61752-3

Manson JE, Greenland P, LaCroix AZ, et al. Walking compared with vigorous exercise for the prevention of cardiovascular events in women. *N Engl J Med.* 2002;347(10):716–725. doi:10.1056/NEJMoa021067

Mao GX, Cao YB, Lan XG, et al. Therapeutic effect of forest bathing on human hypertension in the elderly. *J Cardiol.* 2012;60(6):495–502. doi:10.1016/j.jjcc.2012.08.003

Martland R, Mondelli V, Gaughran F, Stubbs B. Can high-intensity interval training improve physical and mental health outcomes? A meta-review of 33 systematic reviews across the lifespan. *J Sports Sci.* 2020;38(4):430–469. doi:10.1080/02640414.2019.1706829

Moore SC, Lee IM, Weiderpass E, et al. Leisure-time physical activity and risk of 26 types of cancer in 1.44 million adults. *JAMA Intern Med.* 2016;176(6):816–825.

Morris JN, Hardman AE. Walking to health [published correction appears in Sports Med 1997 Aug;24(2):96]. *Sports Med.* 1997;23(5):306–332. doi:10.2165/00007256-199723050-00004

Mosca L. Guidelines for prevention of cardiovascular disease in women: A summary of recommendations. *Prev Cardiol.* 2007;10(Suppl 4):19–25. doi:10.1111/j.1520-037x.2007.07255.x

Mozaffarian D, Benjamin EJ, Go AS, et al. Heart disease and stroke statistics—2015 update: A report from the American Heart Association. *Circulation.* 2015;131:e29–e322.

Overdorf V, Kollia B, Makarec K, Alleva Szeles C. The relationship between physical activity and depressive symptoms in healthy older women. *Gerontol Geriatr Med.* 2016;2:2333721415626859.

Peckham S, Duinker PN, Ordóñez C. Urban forest values in Canada: Views of citizens in Calgary and Halifax. *Urban For. Urban Green.* 2013;12(2):154–162. doi:10.1016/j.ufug.2013.01.001

Piggin J. What is physical activity? A holistic definition for teachers, researchers and policy makers. *Front Sports Act Living.* 2020;2:72. doi:10.3389/fspor.2020.00072

Ross R. Does exercise without weight loss improve insulin sensitivity? *Diabetes Care.* 2003;26(3):944–945. doi:10.2337/diacare.26.3.944

Song C, Ikei H, Kagawa T, Miyazaki Y. Effects of walking in a forest on young women. *Int J Environ Res Public Health.* 2019;16(2):229.

Swain DP, Franklin BA. Comparison of cardioprotective benefits of vigorous versus moderate intensity aerobic exercise. *Am J Cardiol.* 2006;97(1):141–147. doi:10.1016/j.amjcard.2005.07.130

Tsao CW, Vasan RS. The Framingham Heart Study: Past, present and future. *Int J Epidemiol.* 2015;44(6):1763–1766. doi:10.1093/ije/dyv336

Tyrväinen L. Economic valuation of urban forest benefits in Finland. *J Environ Manag.* 2001;62(1):75–92. doi:10.1006/jema.2001.0421

Wang DXM, Yao J, Zirek Y, Reijnierse EM, Maier AB. Muscle mass, strength, and physical performance predicting activities of daily living: A meta-analysis. *J Cachexia Sarcopenia Muscle.* 2020;11(1):3–25. doi:10.1002/jcsm.12502

Warburton DE, Nicol CW, Bredin SS. Health benefits of physical activity: The evidence. *CMAJ.* 2006;174(6):801–809. doi:10.1503/cmaj.051351

Wen Y, Yan Q, Pan Y, Gu X, Liu Y. Medical empirical research on forest bathing (*Shinrin-yoku*): A systematic review. *Environ Health Prev Med*. 2019;24:70. doi:10.1186/s12199-019-0822-8

Woodward M. Cardiovascular disease and the female disadvantage. *Int J Environ Res Public Health*. 2019;16(7):1165. doi:10.3390/ijerp6071165

World Health Organization. *The top 10 causes of death (who.int)*, 2024, 7 August. Retrieved from https://www.who.int/news-room/fact-sheets on 5 September 2024.

Zschucke E, Gaudlitz K, Ströhle A. Exercise and physical activity in mental disorders: Clinical and experimental evidence. *J Prev Med Public Health*. 2013;46(Suppl 1):S12–S21. doi:10.3961/jpmph.2013.46.S.S12

CHAPTER 8

Lifestyle Factors as Contributors to Health Outcomes

8.0 Introduction

Due largely to improvements in sanitation, antibiotics, antivirals, and public immunization programs, deaths caused by infection declined significantly in the 20th and 21st centuries. Although the COVID-19 pandemic brought renewed awareness of the impact of communicable disease on the person, community, and society, we no longer focus on infectious disease as the leading cause of death in developed countries. In fact, even in light of COVID-19, at the time this text was written, most parts of the developed world had returned to normalcy, managing the novel coronavirus, SARS-CoV-2, much like other respiratory viruses. Of course, learning to live with COVID-19 should not distract from the devastation it has caused. As of January 2023, the virus had contributed to 6.69 million deaths worldwide.

Yet the pandemic provided learnings that extended well beyond the realm of infectious diseases, underscoring the importance of health to our civilization and a lack of health equity, locally and globally. The pandemic was sexed, and it was gendered. Epidemiological reports from around the world indicated higher mortality rates in males than females due to biological factors, including sex differences in immunological responses, and attitudinal factors, such as gender differences in willingness to abide by the health measures that were instituted by various authorities for the common good (Bwire, 2020). Other gender disparities were also observed, with women carrying the brunt of the added household, homeschool, and childcare responsibilities during periods of isolation and lockdown and, resultantly, facing reduced income and increased job loss relative to their male colleagues during the pandemic (Dang & Nguyen, 2021). The pandemic exposed the vulnerabilities of marginalized populations, with many minority groups facing disproportionate disease and economic burden in the absence of targeted initiatives. On a further note, events during the years 2020 to 2023 revealed the insufficiency of existing healthcare systems to recognize and respond to the early warning signs of large-scale health emergencies. Examples such as those reported throughout the COVID-19 pandemic highlight the multitude of insights gleaned and

DOI: 10.4324/9781003474777-8

events experienced throughout this period that can be attributed to the belief that what we do affects our health both directly and indirectly.

Indeed, health is reliably linked to behavior at an individual level and at a group level. Our primary focus in healthcare, and especially in achieving positive states of health and well-being, should be centered on behavior as a fundamental aspect of lifestyle. Broadly speaking, lifestyle refers to the way a person lives their life, including the choices, behaviors, and habits they develop and sustain. These factors can significantly affect overall health and well-being, particularly in terms of altering the risk for chronic disease.

According to Pham et al. (2022), non-communicable diseases are the leading causes of death globally and are predicted by a limited set of common, modifiable health behaviors: tobacco use, physical inactivity, harmful use of alcohol, and unhealthy diet. Reports by the WHO concur that 7 of the 10 leading causes of death globally are non-communicable diseases, with cardiovascular disease acting as the world's top killer (WHO, 2020b). Monitoring the leading causes of mortality helps to address their antecedents by adjusting health priorities across multiple sectors, from agriculture (e.g., securing sustainable, affordable healthy foods) to health systems (e.g., prioritizing prevention and early intervention) to public health (e.g., promoting healthy behaviors and reducing harmful behaviors). The death toll of chronic disease highlights a need to focus on lifestyle as an actionable area for improvement to reduce preventable deaths within this domain.

In the U.S., 6 in 10 adults have a chronic disease, and 4 in 10 have two or more chronic diseases. As noted by the U.S. Centers for Disease Control and Prevention (CDC), chronic diseases are defined broadly as conditions that last one year or more and require ongoing medical attention and/or limit activities of daily living. Common examples include heart disease, cancer, chronic lung disease, stroke, Alzheimer's disease, diabetes, and chronic kidney disease. Together, these illnesses are the major drivers of the nation's $3.8 trillion expenditures in healthcare costs. In the same vein, the cost of chronic disease in Canada has been estimated to cost the economy $ CA190 billion annually, with $ CA122 billion in indirect income and productivity losses and $68 billion in direct healthcare costs (CDPAC, 2018).

Chronic diseases are often considered lifestyle diseases because the causes and progressions of the diseases can be attributed to our behaviors (Al-Maskari, 2010). We must ask the question: how can we effect change in the world by changing life conditions and lifestyles toward a health perspective? Further, we must ask this question from a place of non-judgment that aims to meet people where they are to encourage progress and eliminate stigma that can arise in addressing health-related behaviors and decisions. Only in this way will we build autonomy in individuals and communities and reduce reliance on the medical system to manage health.

8.1 Vaccines, Vaccine Confidence, and the Impact of Immunization Programs

Let us continue our discussion of lifestyle and health by considering health behaviors that we can actively control. Consider the development and administration of safe and effective vaccines in protecting people against COVID-19. Several different approaches to vaccinating against SARS-CoV-2 exist. Viral vector vaccines use a harmless virus as a delivery system or "vector." In the case of COVID-19 vaccines, the vector is a modified adenovirus – the same virus that causes the common cold – that contains instructions for producing the SARS-CoV-2 spike protein (i.e., the protein on the surface of the virus that causes COVID-19). Through this process, the protein primes the immune system to produce antibodies and activate other immune cells that will attack SARS-CoV-2 if the virus is encountered. Protein subunit vaccines contain protein pieces of the virus that causes COVID-19 as well as an ingredient called an adjuvant that enhances the immune system's response to the spike protein. Much like viral vector vaccines, once the immune system learns how to attack the spike protein, it will be prepared to respond appropriately if infected with the virus that causes COVID-19. On the other hand, mRNA vaccines contain synthetic genetic material that teaches human cells how to make pieces of spike protein that trigger an immune response to SARS-CoV-2. The genetic material does not enter the cell nucleus, so it cannot be integrated into our own genetic material. Vaccination with any of these vaccines confers protection against COVID-19 without the risks associated with being exposed to the live virus and becoming ill.

As we have discussed in earlier chapters, COVID-19 has stifled multiple areas of life: work, relationships, health service delivery, food production and delivery, and the economy to name a few. The degree of disruption caused by a simple virus emphasizes the need for active and aggressive approaches for containing the pathogen and managing our health amidst raging numbers of new infections. This includes widespread and equitable distribution of approved vaccines to the global population.

If we look to the literature on other illnesses and vaccines, we see that the risk of death and infirmity from diseases such as measles, polio, tuberculosis, diphtheria, and rubella has been largely eliminated when the population participates in public-health immunization programs (Burton, 2002). As Orenstein and Ahmed (2017) stated, the impact in the United States of immunization against vaccine-preventable diseases can be highlighted by comparing representative case numbers in the 20th century with current-day recordings (see Table 8.1 for comparative rates of morbidity for nine infectious diseases). All of these diseases have been reduced by more than 90%, and many have been reduced by 99%. In addition to saving lives, vaccination has resulted in net economic benefits amounting to almost $69 billion in the

Table 8.1 Morbidity of Transmissible Diseases in the U.S. in the 20th Century Relative to 2016, With Percent Decreases

Disease	20th Century Annual Morbidity	2016 Reported Cases	Percent Decrease
Smallpox	29,005	0	100
Diphtheria	21,053	0	100
Measles	539,217	69	>99
Mumps	162,344	5,311	97
Pertussis	200,752	15,737	92
Paralytic polio	16,316	0	100
Rubella	47,745	5	>99
Tetanus	580	33	94
Haemophilus influenzae	20,000	22	>99

Source: Table adapted from Orenstein and Ahmed (2017).

United States alone. Recent cost-savings analyses for 94 low- and middle-income countries estimated that an investment of $34 billion in immunization programs resulted in savings of $586 billion in reducing costs of illness – that's a 17-fold increase in economic gain! Few public health measures have had such a profound impact on society.

Recently, the World Health Organization identified vaccine hesitancy as one of the greatest threats to public health (WHO, 2020b). To address the issue of vaccine hesitancy, we must educate individuals and populations about the science behind disease and immunization. A lack of education may deter individuals from vaccinating due to gaps in knowledge about the effectiveness and safety of vaccines or due to inflexible anti-vaccine attitudes. Indeed, health knowledge in general is associated with more favorable attitudes toward vaccination (Vikram et al., 2012). Vaccines not only provide individual protection for those persons who are vaccinated, they can also provide community protection by reducing the spread of disease within a population. Person-to-person infection is spread when a transmitting case encounters a susceptible person. If the transmitting case only comes in contact with individuals who are immune, then the infection does not spread beyond the index case and is rapidly controlled within the population. Interestingly, this chain of human-to-human transmission can be interrupted even if there is not 100% immunity, because transmitting cases do not have infinite contacts; this is referred to as herd immunity or community protection and is an important benefit of vaccination. Public communications geared at informing individuals of personal and herd immunity may sway public opinions in favor of making decisions about immunization that positively affect health.

8.2 Diet and Nutrition as Modifiable Lifestyle Factors

Another aspect of lifestyle with far-reaching implications for individual and societal health is diet, or the food choices we make and nutritional habits we form. Although there are no randomized controlled trials directly linking sugar consumption to cardiovascular disease, there are several reasons documented in the epidemiological literature why sugar consumption should be limited. For instance, a study by Malik et al. (2019) examined the health effects of long-term consumption of sugar-sweetened beverages and artificially sweetened beverages in U.S. adults. What they found was that intake of sugar-sweetened beverages positively correlated with total mortality, wherein a graded association was observed for cardiovascular disease mortality and a modest association was observed for cancer mortality. Artificially sweetened beverages were positively associated with total disease mortality and cardiovascular disease mortality but not cancer mortality, with stronger associations occurring among women – possibly due to different rates of consumption, metabolic differences, or other interacting factors.

Diets high in added sugars are also known to contribute to type 2 diabetes and Alzheimer's disease. There is robust evidence for the role of dietary sugars, such as fructose and sucrose, in the development of type 2 diabetes, and recent research has documented connections between type 2 diabetes and Alzheimer's disease. For instance, type 2 diabetes and Alzheimer's disease share similar patient profiles, risk factors, and clinical features, such as insulin resistance. Further, being diagnosed with type 2 diabetes is a strong risk factor for developing cognitive impairment in general and Alzheimer's disease more specifically (Cholerton et al., 2016). Given the predisposing role of high-sugar diets in the pathogenesis of both diseases, dietary recommendations aimed at reducing sugar consumption may have preventative value in reducing rates of these two chronic conditions, improving the health and quality of life of large sectors of the population (Moreira, 2013).

According to the Chronic Disease Prevention Alliance of Canada (CDPAC, 2018), sugary drinks are the greatest contributor of sugar in North American diets, and as we have seen, sugar is a prominent driver of chronic disease. Numerous health organizations and political authorities have suggested a need to control consumption of sugary drinks through public health policy to encourage people to make healthier choices. In Canada, it has been projected that sugary drink consumption will be responsible for almost 1 million cases of type 2 diabetes and roughly 300,000 cases of ischemic heart disease over the next 25 years (Jones et al., 2017). This same report, sanctioned by leading health organizations across the country, suggested that a 20% excise levy on the manufacturers of sugary drinks would prevent up to 200,000 cases of type 2 diabetes, avert over 60,000 cases of ischemic heart disease, and result in 13,000 preventable deaths over a 25-year period.

The regular consumption of high-sugar beverages comes not only with a toll to our health but with significant economic costs. In Canada, the healthcare costs attributed to diet-related disease has been estimated at $26 billion/annum. As calculated in the Jones et al. report, a 20% levy on sugary drinks would lead to a total of $11.5 billion in healthcare savings and would generate government revenue of $1.7 billion per year over the 25-year projection period. Based on the findings of this Canadian health research report, the Chronic Disease Prevention Alliance of Canada presented a recommendation to the Canadian House of Commons on Finance in support of such a levy. Further, a 2017 survey commissioned by the Canadian Heart and Stroke Foundation found that approximately 70% of surveyed Canadians are supportive of a levy on companies that make sugary drinks if some of the corresponding revenue is devoted to healthy-living initiatives.

Other approaches aimed at curbing sugary drink consumption have centered on reducing beverage size, with one of the most public examples of this being former New York City Mayor Bloomberg's "soda ban." The sugary drinks portion cap rule, also referred to as the soda ban, was strongly supported by Michael Bloomberg as well as by the NYC Board of Health and was intended to prohibit sale of sugary drinks that were over 16 ounces in size at food service establishments, such as restaurants, delis, movie theaters, sports stadiums, and food carts. Although the regulatory policy was strongly supported by its proponents, in June of 2014, the New York Court of Appeals ruled that the policy fell outside of the New York City Board of Health's scope of authority.

In 2015, the World Health Organization held a technical meeting on Fiscal Policies for Diet and Prevention of Noncommunicable Diseases to address a growing number of requests by policymakers around the globe for guidance on how to design fiscal policies regarding diet. The meeting presented content from the Global Action Plan for the Prevention and Control of Noncommunicable Diseases, proposing that, as appropriate to national contexts, stakeholders consider the use of economic tools to improve access to healthy dietary choices and discourage the consumption of less healthy options. Evidence discussed at the meeting supported the use of taxes and other fiscal policies to reduce consumption of unhealthy foods – in particular, sugar-sweetened beverages – especially if retail prices were raised by 20% or more. Similarly, evidence was presented on encouraging consumption of healthy foods, such as fruits and vegetables, by reducing their prices by 10% to 30%. Although there are different political and public views regarding whether food choices are a matter of public policy or personal autonomy, it is clear that there is a need for change if we are to see a reduction in dietary-related chronic diseases. Whether consumption is controlled through government policy or through initiatives aimed at supporting individuals to make healthier choices, something must be done to curb sugar intake and mitigate its adverse health consequences.

8.3 Physical Inactivity and Sedentary Behavior as Leading Risk Factors for Non-Communicable Illness

Physical inactivity is one of the foremost risks for non-communicable disease mortality. People who are insufficiently active have as much as a 30% increase in risk of early mortality compared to people who are sufficiently active. In combination with other lifestyle factors, such as achieving a healthy weight, eating a healthy diet, and avoiding smoking, exercise can reduce the risk of developing a chronic disease by up to 80% (Al-Maskari, 2010). Yet despite the well-known benefits of exercise and living a physically active lifestyle, only a small percentage of adults engage in regular physical activity.

According to the Centers for Disease Control, physical activity guidelines for Americans include 150 minutes of moderate-intensity physical activity each week, which can be broken down into smaller segments, such as 30 minutes of activity five times a week (Piercy et al., 2018). These recommendations dovetail with the most recent guidelines on physical activity released by the World Health Organization. However, globally, an estimated 28% of adults aged 18 and over do not meet these recommended guidelines. In high-income countries, the percentage of adults who are insufficiently active is slightly higher, at 26% for men and 35% for women. Metrics for adolescent physical activity are even more concerning, with 80% of the global adolescent population falling short of the recommended 60 minutes of physical activity per day (WHO, 2020b). Given that lifelong habits are formed in childhood and adolescence, there is a need for targeted programs that promote physical activity in these stages of development to promote health and longevity in future generations of adults. Although at first blush, exercise may be viewed as a personal practice, the noted statistics highlight physical inactivity as a large-scale social issue that would best be addressed as a public health matter.

A lifestyle factor related to but distinct from physical exercise is the amount of time a person spends engaged in sedentary behavior. In general, our lives are becoming increasingly sedentary with the regular use of motor vehicles for transportation and electronics for work, leisure, and learning. Sedentary behavior can be operationalized as the amount of daily time spent sitting (Matthews et al., 2008). However, more specific definitions have been developed that address both energy expenditure requirements (less than or equal to 1.5 METS) and postural requirements (sitting, reclining, or lying; Tremblay et al., 2017). A MET, or metabolic equivalent, is the ratio of working metabolic rate relative to resting (or basal) metabolic rate, and is based on the amount of oxygen consumption required in both states. A MET of close to 1 is typically obtained during quiet sitting. According to these definitions, children and adults in the U.S. spend approximately 55% of their waking hours being sedentary (Matthews et al., 2008).

Excessive sedentary behavior has been associated with specific disease profiles. In children and youth, too much time engaged in sedentary behavior increases adiposity, impairs cardiometabolic function, and predicts poor sleep quality (WHO, 2020b). In adults, sedentary behavior has been associated with all-cause mortality, cardiovascular disease mortality and incidence of cardiovascular disease, type 2 diabetes, and endometrial, colon, and lung cancer (Katzmarzyk et al., 2019). Importantly, this new perspective on the deleterious health effects of too much sitting should be seen as being additional to and not as an alternative to the well-recognized benefits of participation in moderate-intensity physical activity. In other words, not only should we strive for the advised amount of physical activity each day, we should also aim to limit the amount of time spent sitting. As we have seen, limiting excessive time spent sitting would reduce the population health burden and early mortality associated with major forms of chronic disease, such as type 2 diabetes, cardiovascular disease, and specified forms of cancer (Katzmarzyk et al., 2019).

8.4 Sleep, Sleep Deprivation, and Sleep Hygiene

Sleep occupies almost a third of our life and, thus, is an important aspect of our existence. Sleep deprivation not only disrupts how we function cognitively, emotionally, and physically, but also contributes to common mental health problems, including depression (Ban & Lee, 2001). In fact, although sleep disturbances are a core symptom of depression, they are also an antecedent to mental illness, increasing the risk of clinical depression three- to fivefold. A recent study published in the journal *Sleep* found that sleep deprivation at baseline, defined as 6 or fewer hours of sleep per night, predicted depression at one-year follow-up, controlling for depressive symptomology at baseline (Roberts & Duong, 2014).

Sleep disturbances are common among university students and have an effect on this group's overall health and functioning. The pressures of academic workload and achieving good grades, along with coexisting interpersonal and financial stressors, can affect lifestyle in a number of ways, including the amount and quality of sleep one gets. Assaad and colleagues investigated sleep habits and disorders in a population of university students across Lebanon. Results indicated that only about half of participants were considered "good sleepers," according to their scores on a sleep quality scale, and males experienced more sleep difficulties than females. Further, poor sleep quality was strongly associated with daytime dysfunction and the use of sleep-enhancing medications, many of which have potentially serious side effects.

A significant amount of research has been devoted to addressing the issue of sleep and sleep pathology, spanning disciplines of medicine, neuroscience, psychology, and psychiatry and resulting in solid guidelines for good sleep hygiene. Sleep hygiene includes both behavioral and environmental components and can contribute to better quality sleep and improved overall health.

Establishing a regular schedule for bedtimes and wake-up times normalizes sleep as part of your daily routine and contributes to more regular circadian rhythms. Creating a nightly routine, such as listening to soft music, putting on your pajamas, and brushing your teeth, can generate consistency and help signal to the body and brain that it is time for sleep. Dimming the lights can contribute to better sleep quality, possibly through neurophysiological mechanisms, such as upregulated melatonin production triggered by a darker environment (Lewy et al., 1980). Experts agree that having a window of time before bed away from electronics, such as cell phones, tablets, laptops, and TVs, helps limit cognitive stimulation and encourages melatonin production, both of which may contribute to sleep success (Irish et al., 2015).

Notably, it is not just nighttime habits that contribute to sleep quality. Rather, making changes throughout the day, such as getting enough natural light exposure, being physically active, and limiting caffeine intake can all have lasting effects that translate into better sleep. Finally, finding ways to cope with stress and encourage relaxation, such as journaling, breathwork, mindfulness meditations, and other techniques, can inspire the right mindset for sleep. Communication and implementation of these sleep hygiene recommendations have both clinical and public health implications (Irish et al., 2015).

> ### Avoiding the use of alcohol, tobacco, and other substances promotes health and reduces disease risk.

Alcohol increases the risk of a number of chronic illnesses, including a range of cancers. The UK Committee on Carcinogenicity (COC) released a statement in 2015 advising of the increased risk of cancer of the mouth, throat, larynx, bowel, liver, breast, and pancreas in individuals who consume alcohol. This COC document echoed prior research led by the World Health Organization's International Agency for Research on Cancer (IARC), which clearly documented links between alcohol consumption and a variety of cancers in men and women. These health risks associated with alcohol use are reflected in Canada's new guidelines on alcohol and health, which were released in January 2023. In short, the guidelines emphasize a continuum of risk associated with weekly alcohol use, highlighting the health benefits of abstaining from alcohol. Two drinks or less per week is considered a threshold for low-risk drinking in the new recommendations, whereby alcohol-related harms are deemed to be unlikely at this level of consumption. Three or more drinks per week, on the other hand, is reported to increase the risk of several types of cancer, including breast and colon cancer, whereas seven or more drinks is tied to significant increases in the likelihood of heart disease and stroke. These guidelines are presented with the understanding that a standard drink is 17.05 millilitres of pure alcohol, which is the equivalent of a bottle of beer, a glass of wine, or a shot of spirits. The bottom line? When it comes to alcohol and health, less is better.

These new Canadian guidelines diverge noticeably from earlier national low-risk drinking guidelines, which listed 10 drinks a week for women and 15 drinks a week for men as the cut-off for managing health risks associated with alcohol use. The 2023 Canadian guidance also deviates from current guidelines in other countries, such as the UK, which advises men and women to refrain from drinking more than 14 units of alcohol per week, and the U.S., which advises adults of legal drinking age not to drink or to drink in moderation by limiting intake to 2 drinks or less per day for men or 1 drink or less per day for women (Dietary Guidelines for Americans, 2020). In Canada, scaling down the low-risk threshold will mean updating alcohol policy, public health resources, and medical advice concerning alcohol and health. With emerging knowledge on the harms of regular alcohol use, time will tell whether other countries take a cue from Canada and impose stricter guidance regarding alcohol use in an attempt to reduce the associated risk of morbidity and mortality.

Smoking is the leading cause of preventable morbidity and mortality in America and worldwide. In 2018, U.S. tobacco companies spent $9.06 billion marketing cigarettes and smokeless tobacco. This amount translates to about $25 million each day or more than $1 million every hour. By comparison, smoking-related diseases (i.e., COPD, lung cancer, emphysema, heart disease) cost the United States more than $300 billion each year, which includes approximately $170 billion to cover the direct medical care for adults along with $156 billion that can be attributed to lost productivity directly and a further $5.6 billion that is associated with lost productivity due to exposure to second hand smoke (Action on Smoking and Health, 2020). Initially, vaping was presented as a solution to the massive health consequences of smoking, with e-cigarette companies touting these products as a safer alternative. However, recent research disputes these claims, emphasizing that vaping is not the answer.

E-cigarettes heat nicotine (extracted from tobacco), flavorings, and other chemicals to create an aerosol that is inhaled. Vaping exposes people to harmful chemicals, like formaldehyde and acrolein, and metals and other contaminants, like nickel, tin, and aluminum, many of which are known carcinogens and irritants. Vegetable glycerin and propylene glycol are used as filler liquids in vaping products. While these are considered safe for use in many consumer products, such as cosmetics and sweeteners, the long-term safety of inhaling the substances in vaping products is unknown and continues to be assessed.[1] A large-scale National Health and Nutrition Examination Survey in the U.S. compared cancer prevalence in cigarette smokers, e-cigarette smokers, and non-smokers and found that vaping is associated with earlier onset of cancer compared to traditional smoking, and vaping increases the chance of developing a number of forms of cancer relative to non-smokers (Chidharla et al., 2022).

Views on cannabis and health tend to be dichotomized – that is, people either demonize cannabis use and its presence in society, or they glorify it. What has been shown however is that cannabis is not a panacea, nor will it cause serious problems for everyone who uses it. Cannabis has two distinct psychoactive components – THC (tetrahydrocannabinol) and cannabidiol (CBD). Typically, higher-potency products, that is products with higher THC content, are associated with greater health risks, including mental health risks such as cannabis-related psychosis (Di Forti et al., 2009). This is of significant concern given the steady rise in THC content over recent decades and the normalized use of edibles, which commonly contain 5 to 10 mg of THC (Hudson & Hudson, 2021). Along with documented mental health harms, smoking cannabis is also associated with airway inflammation, chronic bronchitis, increased risk of developing respiratory infections, and, potentially, increased susceptibility for respiratory cancers based on the presence of carcinogenic byproducts, although there is a need for conclusive research in this area (NIDA, 2019). From a medicinal perspective, cannabis is approved for prescribing purposes for a limited number of conditions (e.g., pain/spasticity in multiple sclerosis; nausea in patients undergoing chemotherapy), and there remains considerable controversy over prescribing cannabis for mental health conditions, such as PTSD or anxiety (Schlag et al., 2021). Clearly, there is a need for public education and improved health literacy to correct misperceived risks and benefits of cannabis among the public.

8.5 Conclusion

A person's lifestyle has a substantial impact on their health and life expectancy. By making healthy lifestyle choices, such as getting vaccinated, eating a healthy diet, getting sufficient physical activity, practicing good sleep hygiene, and limiting or avoiding alcohol and other substances, a person can gain control of their health and increase their chances of living a long and vibrant life. Notably, introducing lifestyle changes requires both knowledge of health-promoting and health-impeding behaviors as well as the motivation and ability to implement that knowledge to make the necessary behavioral changes. This concept of modifiable behavior and the vast impact it could have on the leading causes of morbidity and mortality, once again, underscores the need for a holistic approach to health that incorporates theory and expertise from multiple disciplines and professions.

8.5.1 Discussion Questions

1   As noted in this chapter, health and well-being are reliably linked to behaviors at an individual level as well as at a group level. In what ways can we promote positive behaviors as fundamental aspects of our lifestyle?

2   Avoiding specific behaviors, or at least considering moderation as a control mechanism to maintain or achieve positive states of health and well-being, is recognized throughout the related literature. Discuss the influence of health literacy, stigma, and the various determinants of health on behaviors that are recognized antagonists to achieving positive states of health and well-being.

Note

1 Retrieved from Risks of vaping – Canada.ca July 2024.

References

Action on Smoking and Health. (2020). Tobacco control in the United States: Failure to protect the right to health. *Tobacco Prevention & Cessation, 6*, 34. doi:10.18332/tpc/122543. PMID: 32760868; PMCID: PMC7398129.

Al-Maskari, F. (2010). Lifestyle diseases: An economic burden on the health services. *UN Chronicle: The Magazine of the United Nations, 5*, 1–2.

Ban, D. J., & Lee, T. J. (2001). Sleep duration, subjective sleep disturbances and associated factors among University Students in Korea. *Journal of Korean Medical Science, 16*(4), 475–480.

Burton, D. R. (2002). Antibodies, viruses and vaccines. *Nature Reviews Immunology, 2*, 706–713.

Bwire, G. M. (2020). Coronavirus: Why men are more vulnerable to Covid-19 than women? *SN Comprehensive Clinical Medicine, 2*(7), 874–876.

Chidharla, A., Agarwal, K., Abdelwahed, S., Bhandari, R., Singh, A., Rabbani, R., . . . Koritala, T. (2022). Cancer prevalence in E-cigarette users: A retrospective cross-sectional NHANES study. *World Journal of Oncology, 13*(1), 20.

Cholerton, B., Baker, L. D., Montine, T. J., & Craft, S. (2016). Type 2 diabetes, cognition, and dementia in older adults: Toward a precision health approach. *Diabetes Spectrum. 29*(4), 210–219. doi:10.2337/ds16-0041

Chronic Disease Prevention Alliance of Canada (CDPAC). (2018). Pre-budget submission to the House of Commons Standing Committee on Finance, 4 August 2017. Retrieved on 4 September 2024.

Dang, H. A. H., & Nguyen, C. V. (2021). Gender inequality during the COVID-19 pandemic: Income, expenditure, savings, and job loss. *World Development, 140,* 105296.

Di Forti, M., Morgan, C., Dazzan, P., Pariante, C., Mondelli, V., Marques, T. R., . . . & Murray, R. M. (2009). High-potency cannabis and the risk of psychosis. *The British Journal of Psychiatry, 195*(6), 488–491.

Hudson, A., & Hudson, P. (2021). Risk factors for cannabis-related mental health harms in older adults: A review. *Clinical Gerontologist, 44*(1), 3–15.

Irish, L. A., Kline, C. E., Gunn, H. E., Buysse, D. J., & Hall, M. H. (2015). The role of sleep hygiene in promoting public health: A review of empirical evidence. *Sleep Medicine Reviews, 22,* 23–36.

Jones, A. C., Veerman, J. L., & Hammond, D. (2017, April). The health and economic impact of a tax on sugary drinks in Canada (technical teport). Retrieved from http://www.2017-sugary-drink-tax-provincial-estimates-reports-alberta-final.pdf (abpolicycoalitionforprevention.ca) (accepted 4 September 2024).

Katzmarzyk, P. T., Powell, K. E., Jakicic, J. M., Troiano, R. P., Piercy, K., Tennant, B., & 2018 Physical Activity Guidelines Advisory Committee. (2019). Sedentary behavior and health: Update from the 2018 physical activity guidelines advisory committee. *Medicine and Science in Sports and Exercise, 51*(6), 1227.

Lewy, A. J., Wehr, T. A., Goodwin, F. K., Newsome, D. A., & Markey, S. P. (1980). Light suppresses melatonin secretion in humans. *Science, 210,* 1267–1269.

Malik, V. S., Li, Y., Pan, A., De Koning, L., Schernhammer, E., Willett, W. C., & Hu, F. B. (2019). Long-term consumption of sugar-sweetened and artificially sweetened beverages and risk of mortality in US adults. *Circulation, 139*(18), 2113–2125.

Matthews, C. E., Chen, K. Y., Freedson, P. S., Buchowski, M. S., Beech, B. M., Pate, R. R., & Troiano, R. P. (2008). Amount of time spent in sedentary behaviors in the United States, 2003–2004. *American Journal of Epidemiology, 167,* 875–881.

Moreira, P. I. (2013). High-sugar diets, type 2 diabetes and Alzheimer's disease. *Current Opinion in Clinical Nutrition & Metabolic Care, 16*(4), 440–445.

National Institute on Drug Abuse. (2019). *Cannabis drug facts.* Retrieved on 9 September 2024.

Orenstein, W. A., & Ahmed, R. (2017). Simply put: Vaccination saves lives. *Proceedings of the National Academy of Sciences of the United States of America, 114*(16), 4031–4033. doi:10.1073/pnas.1704507114

Pham, B. N., Jorry, R., Abori, N., Silas, V. D., Okely, A. D., & Pomat, W. (2022). Non-communicable diseases attributed mortality and associated sociodemographic factors in Papua New Guinea: Evidence from the Comprehensive Health and Epidemiological Surveillance System. *PLOS Global Public Health, 2*(3). https://doi.org/10.1371/journal.pgph.0000118

Piercy, K. L., Troiano, R. P., Ballard, R. M., Carlson, S. A., Fulton, J. E., Galuska, D. A., . . . Olson, R. D. (2018). The physical activity guidelines for Americans. *JAMA, 320*(19), 2020–2028.

Roberts, R. E., & Duong, H. T. (2014). The prospective association between sleep deprivation and depression among adolescents. *Sleep, 37*(2), 239–244.

Schlag, A. K., O'Sullivan, S. E., Zafar, R. R., & Nutt, D. J. (2021). Current controversies in medical cannabis: Recent developments in human clinical applications and potential therapeutics. *Neuropharmacology, 191,* 108586.

Tremblay, M. S., Aubert, S., Barnes, J. D., Saunders, T. J., Carson, V., Latimer-Cheung, A. E., . . . Chinapaw, M. J. M. (2017). Sedentary Behavior Research Network (SBRN) – Terminology consensus project process and outcome. *International Journal of Behavioral Nutrition and Physical Activity, 14*(1), 75.

U.S. Department of Agriculture and U.S. Department of Health and Human Services. (2020, December). *Dietary guidelines for Aamericans, 2020–2025.* 9th edition. Available at DietaryGuidelines.gov.

Vikram, K., Vanneman, R., & Desai, S. (2012). Linkages between maternal education and childhood immunization in India. *Social Science & Medicine, 75,* 331–339.

World Health Organization. (2020a). *Global health estimates: Deaths by cause, age, sex, by country and by region, 2000–2019.* Geneva: Global Health Estimates: Leading Causes of Death (who. int). Retrieved from https://www.who.int/data/gho/data/themes/mortality-and-global-health-estimates on 5 September 2024.

World Health Organization. (2020b). *WHO guidelines on physical activity and sedentary behavior.* Geneva: World Health Organization. Licence: CC BY-NC-SA 3.0 IGO. Retrieved from https://www.who.int/publications/i/item/9789240015128 on 5 September 2024.

CHAPTER 9

Mental Health and Addictions

9.0 Introduction

In keeping with the World Health Organization's definition of health, outlined in Chapter 1, we will define mental health as more than the absence of a psychiatric disorder or illness and, instead, frame it as a state of mental well-being determined by many interrelated factors. When we take this type of holistic perspective, we acknowledge that although 1 in 5 individuals experience mental illness within any given year, 5 in 5 have mental health and can take steps to improve their mental health.

Indeed, mental health can be broadly defined as the capacity of each and all of us to feel, think, and act in ways that support our ability to have a meaningful life and to cope effectively with challenges (Public Health Agency of Canada, 2017). In contrast, mental illness can be described as patterns of cognition, emotion, and behavior that cause significant distress to the individual and/or notable impairment to their daily functioning (Canadian Mental Health Association, 2020). When we compare these definitions of mental health and mental illness, we see that they are not dichotomous, nor are they opposite ends of the same spectrum. Lacking a diagnosis of a mental illness does not necessarily guarantee good mental health. In the same way, an individual may have a psychiatric illness but be managing symptoms and attaining high levels of mental well-being.

Definitions of mental health may vary from one individual or group to another, but there are six common elements of mental well-being that are emphasized in definitions from across Canada and around the world: a sense of purpose, strong interpersonal relationships, feelings of connectedness to others, a strong sense of self, an ability to cope with stress, and a capacity to enjoy life.

9.1 Cross-Cultural Conceptualizations of Mental Health and Illness

The way we identify and explain mental disorders across cultures and contexts is not always analogous. How individuals understand mental health is strongly rooted in their

DOI: 10.4324/9781003474777-9

cultural beliefs and is predictive of the ways in which they aim to treat or heal from mental illness (Sheikh & Furnham, 2000). In non-Western cultures, underlying beliefs about mental illness tend to revolve around supernatural causes (i.e., the will of God, violation of social or religious rituals), whereas in Western society, explanations are geared toward natural causes (i.e., neurochemical imbalances) or personal issues (stress, lifestyle). Non-Western cultures also view physiological factors as determinants of health but may subscribe to alternate causative factors, such as heat in the body, imbalances in the body, or currents of wind or gas in the body (Eisenbruch, 1990).

Anthropological studies on the origins and manifestation of mental illness reveal a number of important disparities across cultures. In a survey-based study about disease etiology, Asians were found to endorse supernatural, Western, and non-Western physiological explanations of mental illness (Sheikh & Furnham, 2000). In the same study, Muslims scored high on supernatural causes of mental illness, seeing mental suffering as attributable to religiosity and religious practices. Pakistanis exhibited pluralistic beliefs, endorsing both Western and non-Western viewpoints. Such cultural beliefs can play a role in determining help-seeking behaviors, such as relying on prayer in cases where supernatural causes are believed to be at play or taking psychoactive medication in cases where chemical imbalances are the suspected source of the ailment. Whether mental health problems should be addressed at church or one's place of worship, in a formal healthcare setting, or both is, thus, largely culturally dependent.

The prevalence and presentation of mental illness can also vary widely from one culture to another. Let us consider depression as an example. Epidemiological research conducted as part of the global burden of disease study has shown that over 5% of the population has a clinical depression diagnosis in the Middle East, North Africa, sub-Saharan Africa, Eastern Europe, and the Caribbean. Meanwhile, depression is reportedly lowest, affecting less than 2% of the population, in East Asia, followed by Australia/New Zealand and Southeast Asia (Ferrari et al., 2013). According to the researchers who led this report, countries with the highest rates of depression are characterized by high levels of war or conflict and the presence of other collective stressors, such as public health epidemics, high unemployment rates, and extreme wealth inequity. It is important to note that rates reported in this study do not necessarily reflect true rates of clinical depression so much as the rate at which people are diagnosed with the disorder. Countries with poor mental health awareness or resources may show misleadingly low rates (e.g., Iraq). Regions where mental illness continues to be taboo (e.g., East Asia) may have disproportionately low rates due to an unwillingness to seek help for mental health concerns.

We have considered global differences in the prevalence of mental illness; now, let us examine cultural disparities in the presentation of mental illness. For instance, depression may look different in individualistic cultures, such as the United States or Canada, than in collectivist cultures, such as those observed in Japan or China. In Asian countries, where society values community, selflessness, and altruism, it is more common to report somatic symptoms of depression (i.e., headaches, lack of sleep), perhaps because it is culturally expected to suppress emotional symptoms (i.e., prolonged sadness). In Western cultures, on the other hand, where personal identity is prioritized, emotional symptoms predominate, and somatic symptoms are less frequently reported as the chief complaint. Depression as a disease entity is entirely missing in other cultures. Many Indigenous languages do not have specific terms for depression or may use alternate words and phrases to explain similar conditions. This is not to say that depression does not exist among these populations but, rather, that it is expressed and understood differently.

Understanding cultural narratives of mental illness is imperative, as it shapes how care providers assess and treat patients from different backgrounds. Furthermore, there are virtually no cross-cultural adaptations of standard diagnostic tools, which makes existing classification practices ill-suited for use in many cultures. A relatively new branch of medicine, known as ethnomedicine, recognizes the importance of culture, perception, and context in shaping mental and physical health. Studies at the intersection of ethnomedicine and mental health hold promise in advancing how we assess and treat mental health issues in a way that is respectful of cultural diversity.

9.2 Diagnosing Mental Illness

Although knowledge of mental illness cannot fully inform our understanding of mental health, it provides context for studying variable cognitive, emotional, and behavioral states. Further, there is value in understanding psychiatric illness to help inform prevention, early intervention, and treatment efforts. Examples of mental or psychiatric disorders include mood disorders, anxiety disorders, psychotic disorders, personality disorders, eating disorders, and substance use disorders. Classification standards for diagnosing mental disorders follow criteria outlined in the *Diagnostic and Statistical Manual of Mental Disorders, 5th Edition* (DSM-5) and require assessment by an authorized healthcare professional. The DSM-5 was published in 2013 – 61 years after the original DSM – and is based on the most recent research and clinical evidence. It contains 20 disorder chapters and nearly 300 mental illnesses. Individuals may display some symptoms but not meet full diagnostic criteria for a particular disorder, introducing a spectrum of mental health issues that range from non-clinical to clinical.

Whereas the DSM-5 is the classification system standardly applied in diagnosing and treating mental illness in North America and Australia, other regions of the world gravitate toward an alternate classification framework, namely the International Classification of Diseases 11th Revision, or the ICD-11. Originating over a century ago, the latest version of the ICD was approved by the 72nd World Health Assembly in 2019 and came into effect in January 2022. The ICD serves a number of purposes, including, but not limited to, collecting data on worldwide causes of morbidity and mortality, recording data on diseases in primary, secondary, and tertiary care settings, and enabling comparative health research across contexts and countries. Among its applications, it also provides clinical descriptions and diagnostic guidelines for 21 broad categories of mental disorders, which are further broken down into specific clinical diagnoses.

During the creation of the DSM-5 and the ICD-11, developers aimed to align the two systems, although separate priorities and mandates of the WHO and APA mean that several differences persist. For instance, the ICD covers all health conditions, both physical and mental, while the DSM focuses solely on mental disorders. The ICD, published by the World Health Organization, is the international standard system for classifying all medical diseases. The DSM is the American Psychiatric Association's standard reference for psychiatry and is applied consistently in North America and Australia and is gaining popularity in terms of international use.

According to reviews aimed at evaluating alignment efforts of the latest versions of the DSM and ICD, the two systems are very similar at the organizational level. Yet there are 19 ICD-11 disorder categories that do not appear in DSM-5 and seven DSM-5 categories that do not appear in the ICD-11. Of the mental disorders that appear in both systems, 31 share identical diagnostic criteria, and 10 other disorders differ only in the degree of specificity, with greater operational specificity presented in the DSM-5 compared to the ICD-11. This represents significant improvements in overlapping interpretation and organization relative to their precursors (First et al., 2021). Although there are some noted disparities between the two aforementioned classification systems, they are both empirical, evidence-based means for representing and organizing mental disorders.

9.3 Common Mental Disorders

Some of the most common mental disorders are mood disorders, including depression and bipolar disorder, anxiety disorders, including generalized anxiety disorder (GAD), panic disorder, specific phobias, and substance use disorders. In epidemiology, prevalence is described as the proportion of a population affected by a condition of interest at a specific point or period in time. It can be captured as point prevalence (proportion affected at a specific time point), period prevalence (proportion affected over the course of a designated time frame, such as a year), or lifetime prevalence (proportion affected during the course of their life). The lifetime prevalence rate for major depressive disorder is 10% to 15%, and rates are slightly higher in women than in men. Comparable lifetime prevalence rates have been documented for generalized anxiety disorder, and comorbidity rates are high at roughly 50% for these two conditions. Lifetime and 12-month prevalence rates for alcohol use disorder are estimated at 30% and 14%, respectively (Grant et al., 2015). Given the pervasiveness of these disorders, and for the sake of brevity, this chapter will focus on major depressive disorder, GAD, and substance use disorders.

Depression is more than just feeling down or having a bad day. However, when a sad mood persists over a long period of time and interferes with everyday functioning, a diagnosis of depression may be warranted. According to the DSM-5, major depressive disorder can be rated as mild, moderate, or severe and can occur with or without psychosis. A diagnosis requires that at least five of the criterion symptoms are present for at least a two-week period, and one of the symptoms must be anhedonia or lack of pleasure or interest. Other symptoms include significant weight change or appetite disturbance, sleep disturbance (insomnia or hypersomnia), psychomotor agitation or retardation, fatigue or loss of energy, feelings of worthlessness or helplessness, cognitive symptoms such as slowed thought processes or indecisiveness, and suicidal ideation or behavior. As with other mental disorders, the symptoms must cause significant distress and impairment and cannot be explained by pharmacological/medical factors or another diagnosis.

Anxiety is experienced on a spectrum from non-clinical to clinical (diagnosable) anxiety. Anxiety and apprehension are normal responses to unpredictable, new, or high-stakes situations. In some cases, anxiety is adaptive in that it may encourage motivation, preparation, and consideration. However, anxiety becomes disordered when feelings of nervousness and worry persist over the course of months and interfere with the individual's ability to function in their daily roles. GAD occurs when worry is excessive (i.e., it is disproportionate to the risk at hand), has been present for at least 6 months, is difficult to control, spans a range of circumstances, topics, or events, and co-presents with other designated symptoms. More precisely, three of the following symptoms must accompany the aforementioned criteria: restlessness, fatigue, difficulty concentrating, irritability, physical symptoms such as muscle aches and soreness, and difficulty falling asleep or staying asleep. As with other psychiatric disorders, the symptoms must cause distress and impaired functioning and cannot be ascribed to substance use or a medical condition.

As with anxiety and depression, substance use falls along a continuum, from harmless or even beneficial use to compulsive or disordered use. Substance use can be conceptualized in a variety of ways. Medical models of addiction describe it as a chronic, relapsing disease, influenced by biology and behavior. Social lenses seek to explain substance use outcomes as a product of sociocultural factors that confer risk or resilience in the individual or group. Psychological definitions emphasize continued compulsive substance use despite experiencing significant consequences as a result of use. Clinicians rely on the DSM-5 to classify substance use disorders using 11 criteria, which include symptoms such as loss of control, preoccupation with obtaining and using the substance, using in larger amounts or for longer periods than intended, using despite significant harms, cravings to use the substance, interference with daily activities and responsibilities, tolerance (requiring more of the substance to get the same effect), and withdrawal (experiencing predictable symptoms upon cessation of use). Substance use disorders may be labeled as mild if two to three symptoms are present, moderate if four or five symptoms occur, and severe if six or more symptoms are observed.

The DSM-5 is fundamental in providing a standardized approach to conceptualizing and diagnosing mental disorders for clinicians and researchers alike; granted, some experts caution, and even criticize, the practice of classifying mental illness in this way. For one, critics suggest that the manual lacks validity because diagnoses lack objective standards and measures. Indeed, although biomarkers have been groundbreaking in confirming medical diagnoses and guiding treatment, they remain relatively insubstantial in the field of psychiatric illness. Further, there is growing consensus that mental disorders are not specific diseases but, instead, are syndromes of heterogeneous symptoms. Such a viewpoint challenges the arbitrary boundaries of diagnostic categories. A related criticism is that the DSM tends to medicalize patterns of behaviors, thoughts, and emotions that may be normal reactions to life events, therefore leading to false positive diagnoses and blurring the margins of normal variability and pathology. On the other hand, some individuals may not meet diagnostic criteria despite experiencing significant distress and meriting clinical intervention. The same criticisms can be directed at classification practices based on the ICD-11. In sum, current diagnostic practices may oversimplify human behavior by reducing complex problems with multifaceted etiologies and manifestations to a limited number of labels and codes. Nonetheless, having a consistent set of symptoms to reference does provide standardization for assessment, care planning, and treatment.

9.4 The Impact of Mental Illness

Mental disorders can have long-term negative effects due to ill-health, lost productivity, reduced quality of life, and, in some cases, early mortality. According to the WHO, people with severe mental disorders have a 10- to 25-year reduction in life expectancy compared to the general population. For instance, mortality rates among people with schizophrenia are 2 to 2.5 times higher than the general population, and mortality rates are 1.8 times higher among people with clinical depression than the general population. Amid the causes of premature death, suicide is one of the most prevalent. Nearly 4,000 Canadians die by suicide each year – an average of almost 11 suicides a day. Suicide is one of the leading causes of death in both men and women from adolescence to middle age. For instance, suicide accounts for 24% of all deaths among 15- to 24-year-olds and 16% of deaths among 25- to 44-year-olds in Canada (Government of Canada, 2019). In Western countries, more than 75% of suicides involve men, but women attempt suicide three to four times more often than men (Statistics Canada, 2017).

The psychosocial impact of suicide on families and communities is immeasurable. However, in an attempt to quantify the burden of suicide and to inform decision-makers and funding bodies of the need for support, health researchers monitor indicators of mortality and morbidity. Mortality has been measured in terms of years of life lost, mortality rates, and by ranking of the leading causes of early mortality. In Canada, suicide results in an estimated 100,000 years of life lost in individuals under 75 in a single year (Statistics Canada, 2017). In the 2016 Global Burden of Disease study, which ranked 264 causes of mortality by location, age, and sex, suicide ranked among the top ten leading causes of death in Europe, high-income Asia, Australasia, and high-income North America (Naghavi, 2019). Disability-adjusted life years (DALYs) considers both years of life lost due to premature mortality (YLLs) and years of life affected by illness or disability (YLDs). One Dutch study found that suicide and attempted suicide were responsible for 90,700 DALYs, positioning suicide 11th in a comprehensive list of diseases, following dementia (rank 10) and preceding breast cancer (rank 12). In examining these outcomes, it is apparent that suicide is a global public health issue and a significant cause of preventable early mortality and morbidity.

9.5 Gender, Ethnicity, and Mental Illness

Mental illness affects people from all backgrounds, genders, social classes, and ethnicities; yet prevalence rates are predictably higher in certain subpopulations. When we consider gender differences in mental disorders, women report anxiety and depression at notably higher rates than men, even though men die by suicide more frequently than women. The reasons behind these gender differences are too complex to adequately capture here, but gender norms around masculinity and stoicism, along with reduced help-seeking behaviors in men, are central to this discussion. Accordingly, WHO surveys reveal that women are the primary users of community-based and primary-care services for mental health concerns, whereas men tend to resist presenting for service until problems escalate to a level requiring emergency or inpatient care. Gender and sexual minorities also experience disproportionate rates of mental disorders, substance use, and suicide risk (Mereish et al., 2014). The U.S. National Survey on Drug Use and Health found that 1 in 3 LGBQ (lesbian, gay, bisexual, queer) adults experienced mental illness in 2015, compared with 1 in 5 heterosexual adults (Hedden et al., 2016). LGBQ youth experience suicidal ideation more frequently than the general young adult population and are over four times more likely to attempt suicide relative to heterosexual youth (Kann et al., 2016). Transgender youth are more likely than cisgender youth to have clinical depression and to engage in suicidal behavior, with as many as 1 in 5 transgender youth having attempted suicide (Reisner et al., 2015). Gender-diverse populations may be at increased risk of mental illness and suicidality given the specific challenges they face, including stress of coming out to friends or family, bullying, lack of appropriate supports, discrimination, stigma, and limited access to gender-informed health services. Sex and gender considerations must be integrated into healthcare in a way that acknowledges these risk factors, respects diversity, and prioritizes equity.

Disparities in mental health outcomes have been observed in other minority groups, including the Black, Indigenous, people of color (BIPOC) community. In Canada, First Nations youth die by suicide 5 to 6 times more frequently than non-Indigenous youth, although there is heterogeneity across First Nations communities (Statistics Canada, 2017). One of the major contributors to these bleak outcomes is the historical trauma Indigenous communities in Canada have sustained through the residential school system. Historical trauma, also referred to as cultural trauma, accumulates over time and across generations and often involves the traumatization of a specific population. A related form of trauma, underrepresented in the literature, is racial trauma. Racial trauma is said to occur when an individual or group witnesses or experiences physical or psychological violence related to their race or ethnicity (Williams et al., 2018). Experiences of racial trauma are common among BIPOC communities and have been linked to increased risk of depression, anxiety, and problematic substance use (Clark et al., 2015). Along with increased exposure to violence, trauma, and discrimination, BIPOC populations may also face reduced access to culturally appropriate and safe care. Culturally safe care respects diverse values, sexual orientations, genders, ethnicities, and religious/spiritual views is sensitive to experiences of historical and racial trauma, and allows people to feel that their healthcare is connected in meaningful ways to their identities and their lives.

9.6 Mental Illness and Comorbid Disorders

Often, the most adverse mental health outcomes are seen for individuals who present with multiple morbidities. Comorbidity of mental health and substance use problems is common in Canada. Health Administrative data indicate that 35.6% of individuals admitted to inpatient mental health facilities in Canada have co-occurring substance use disorders (CIHI, 2013). According to the literature, there are four primary reasons for the high co-occurrence of mental health problems and disordered substance use: (1) individuals use substances to self-medicate for pre-existing mental health concerns (e.g., Khantzian, 1985); (2) substance use leads to mental health problems directly (substance-induced symptoms) or indirectly (substance-related interpersonal challenges or financial problems that cause mental and emotional distress; Patton et al., 2002); (3) mental health problems and substance use co-present due to interrelated factors that confer risk for both mental illness and substance misuse (Stewart et al., 2016); (4) mental illness and substance misuse may exist in a cycle, where comorbidity occurs through mechanisms (1) or (2), but a bidirectional link maintains both disorders (Stewart & Conrod, 2007).

Barriers to accessing the appropriate healthcare are particularly robust for individuals with comorbid disorders, and these individuals often rely on multiple segregated services when they would be better served by an integrative approach to care. Integrating mental health and addictions services has several positive outcomes, including improved access to care and enhanced client experience (Kates et al., 2011). An integrated approach to treating mental health and substance use disorders also fits with a growing recognition among the public of interconnections between mental health and substance use (Hudson et al., 2018).

On the topic of comorbidities, research indicates a common prevalence between mental illness and chronic disease. Individuals with mental disorders such as anxiety, depression, schizophrenia, and bipolar disorder show a high prevalence of chronic coronary heart disease, diabetes, obesity, and chronic obstructive pulmonary disease (COPD). Likewise, individuals with chronic physical diseases have higher-than-normal prevalence rates for certain mental disorders. There are a number of pathways that may lead to the co-emergence of chronic physical health conditions and mental health problems. For instance, interrelated factors (i.e., social determinants of health) may place an individual at risk for both forms of illness. Alternatively, experiences of trauma and, in particular, early adversity may alter neuroimmune function in a way that precipitates both mental illness and chronic health conditions. The study of this interaction between psychological processes, the brain, and the immune system constitutes the field of psychoneuroimmunology, which has grown in popularity over recent years for its ability to explain the impact of psychological stress on immune function. Importantly, individuals experiencing chronic medical conditions alongside mental illness often receive healthcare that is inferior to that of the general population. The majority of deaths of patients with severe mental illness that are due to medical conditions are preventable with more attentive checks for physical illness, medication side effects, and suicide risk screening (WHO, 2015).

9.7 Etiology and the Biopsychosocial Model

The etiology of mental disorders is multifactorial and can best be understood from a biopsychosocial framework whereby biological factors (e.g., genetics, individual differences in neural function), psychological factors (e.g., personality traits, cognitive biases), and social factors (e.g., social determinants of health, exposure to early adversity) interact to shape one's propensity for mental health and mental illness. In line with a precision health approach, the relative contribution of risk factors in determining one's mental health status differs for each individual and is influenced by the presence of protective factors that can garner resilience.

The biopsychosocial lens is well aligned with the traditional diathesis-stress model of disease, wherein the development of mental disorders can be viewed as an interaction between a biological and/or psychological predisposition (i.e., the diathesis) and socioenvironmental conditions or life experiences (i.e., the stressor). To illustrate, consider the finding that although 1 in 5 Canadians are living with a mental illness, 1 in 3 Canadians below the poverty line experience mental illness annually. In this example, we witness the impact of a social issue – low income and the associated consequences of inadequate housing, food insecurity, financial stress, and so on – in shifting the trajectory from health to illness. Yet there is heterogeneity in mental health outcomes for any social demographic, highlighting how biological and psychological predispositions and buffers interact with the social circumstances in which an individual lives to induce health or illness.

The interaction between disposition and stimulus can also be observed in the phenomenon of drug-induced psychosis. Cannabis is a known risk factor for schizophrenia and other psychotic disorders, although the exact process through which cannabis induces psychosis is intricate and not well understood. For instance, it remains unclear why individuals may use cannabis in similar doses and at similar frequencies but show divergent mental health outcomes in terms of susceptibility for psychosis. One school of thought proposes that individuals who develop psychosis or schizophrenia following cannabis use may carry a predisposition that is essentially "turned on" by the psychoactive substance (Tibbo et al., 2018).

9.8 Stigma

Stigma can literally be defined as a mark of disgrace or reproach. Put more elaborately, stigma occurs as a complex social process of labeling, devaluing, and discriminating and operates at various levels within the healthcare sector (Link & Phelan, 2001). Stigma may occur intrapersonally when negative beliefs and attitudes about the particular attribute or condition are held by the individual themself. In this way, intrapersonal stigma involves embodied feelings of guilt, shame, and embarrassment, influencing how a person sees themself, how they relate with others, and, in the case of healthcare, how they seek and receive treatment. Interpersonal stigma, as the name implies, involves negative relationships and interactions with others as a result of a particular attribute or condition. In the case of healthcare, it may involve negative beliefs or attitudes held by care providers regarding a specific condition or patient population, thereby diminishing patient–provider rapport and quality of care provided. Finally, structural stigma occurs at the level of the system or organization and may entail policies, practices, or programming that are discriminatory against a particular condition or patient population. To exemplify, structural stigma may manifest as insufficient allocation of resources to certain services and programs, unwelcoming or judgmental workplace culture, or policies that ignore or marginalize the voice of particular individuals or groups. It is important to note that all of these forms of stigma may be explicit and conscious or may operate more implicitly, without the individual's or system's awareness (Corrigan et al., 2014).

More than any other type of illness, mental illness has been subject to negative judgements and stigmatization. Stigma can be extremely harmful to individuals experiencing mental health challenges, as it can cause further deterioration to their mental health, can lead to feelings of loneliness and worthlessness, and can prevent people from seeking help when it is most needed. Addressing stigma takes understanding, education, and a willingness to examine our own attitudes and language around mental health. A number of evidence-based strategies can be applied to harness acceptance and understanding to reduce stigma historically associated with mental health and addictions. For one, education for healthcare workers and leaders can model person-first healthcare – care that recognizes the individual as a person (as opposed to a patient) who is multifaceted, unique, and able to make decisions about their own healthcare plans. Second, social-contact approaches to stigma reduction engage individuals with lived experience to educate healthcare leaders and clinicians. In this strategy, people with lived experience of mental illness or addiction are seen as experts or educators as opposed to patients. Third, education aimed at correcting myths or fallacies (false beliefs) about mental health and addiction can be transformative in targeting discriminatory attitudes (subconscious or conscious) held by clinicians toward specific patient populations. In sum, interventions geared at emphasizing positive language, correcting misinformation, and lending insight into the experiences and stories of individuals with mental illness can effectively transform health services and systems to alleviate stigma and enhance the safety and quality of care.

9.9 Recovering From Mental Illness

A topic central to the discussion of mental health and mental illness is that of recovery. According to the Substance Abuse and Mental Health Services Administration (SAMHSA), "Recovery from mental health disorders and/or substance use disorders is a process for change through which individuals improve their health and wellness, live a self-directed life and strive to reach their full potential." Other professional organizations, such as the Centre for Addiction and Mental Health (CAMH) and the World Health Organization (WHO), have conceptualized recovery in similar terms. If we subscribe to this definition, then we also recognize that an individual can live with mental illness while still experiencing mental well-being just as someone with diabetes can manage their illness and live a healthy life.

To understand recovery more fully, we should first consider what recovery is not. Recovery is not synonymous with cure. Instead, it encompasses internal conditions, such as hope, healing, and empowerment, and external conditions, such as a social connection, inclusion, and a culture of equity and support. Recovery from mental disorders should not be confused with remission or abstinence (in the case of substance use disorders). A person does not need to be symptom free or substance free to be in recovery. If we held such a reductionist view, recovery would be unattainable for many, and clinicians would be destitute in their attempts to measure progress toward a range of viable goals. For instance, part of recovery for individuals who use substances is often harm reduction, wherein health professionals seek to reduce the negative health and social impacts of substance use without necessarily requiring abstinence or cessation of use. Recovery is not one-size-fits-all but should instead be conceived as a personal journey that centers on an individual's unique circumstances, goals, and strengths. Recovery-oriented professionals meet people where they are and respect the individual's choices and self-determination in navigating their recovery.

It is noteworthy that recovery from mental disorders, which include substance use disorders, can occur with or without professional intervention. In the substance use arena, recovery without formal intervention is often labeled spontaneous or independent recovery. Contrary to what the term *spontaneous* implies, this form of recovery is often a lengthy process involving clear intentions, strong social supports, and numerous changes geared toward a healthier way of being. As many of 60% of individuals who meet criteria for a substance use disorder recover without seeking formal treatment (although this figure would be lower in cases that require medical withdrawal management). Some health researchers and practitioners label this process "maturing out" of problematic substance use, particularly when the population of interest is a younger demographic. As noted, recovery is defined by the individual. For some individuals, this may mean that they choose not to use the term *recovery* to describe their experience.

Instead, improving their mental health and gaining control of their substance use can be seen as a lifestyle change or a commitment to mental and physical wellness. There is literature that suggests that individuals with mild to moderate substance use disorders are less likely to resonate with the term *recovery*.

9.10 Conclusion

Humans are dynamic beings living in complex societies in which biological, psychological, socioeconomic, cultural, and spiritual factors all impact mental health and well-being. Because recovery from mental illness, including substance use disorders, touches families, peers, and communities, and because recovery is multidimensional, it requires collaboration across many different sectors. When we move away from fixating solely on symptoms and substance use and instead emphasize functioning and striving in different life domains, mental well-being becomes attainable for everyone – with or without a mental illness.

9.10.1 Discussion Questions

1   Discuss cultural differences in beliefs about mental health and mental illness. How might cultural beliefs shape prevention and treatment efforts in the domain of mental health and well-being?
2   Define stigma. How does stigma influence mental health? What are some strategies that we might consider to mitigate the effects of stigma? Are there specific cohorts that are more or less impacted by stigma?

References

Canadian Institute for Health Information (CIHI). (2013, March). *Analysis in brief: Hospital mental health services for concurrent mental illness and substance use disorders in Canada.* Retrieved from https://publications.gc.ca/collections/collection_2013/icis-cihi/H117-5-26-2013-eng.pdf (accessed 7 September 2024).

Canadian Mental Health Association. (2020). *Mental health: What is it, really?* https://cmha.ca/mental-health-what-is-it-really/#_ftn1

Clark, T. T., Salas-Wright, C. P., Vaughn, M. G., & Whitfield, K. E. (2015). Everyday discrimination and mood and substance use disorders: A latent profile analysis with African Americans and Caribbean Blacks. *Addictive Behaviors, 40,* 119–125.

Corrigan, P. W., Druss, B. G., & Perlick, D. A. (2014). The impact of mental illness stigma on seeking and participating in mental health care. *Psychological Science in the Public Interest, 15*(2), 37–70. doi:10.1177/1529100614531398

Eisenbruch, M. (1990). Classification of natural and supernatural causes of mental distress. Development of a mental distress explanatory model questionnaire. *The Journal of Nervous and Mental Disease, 178*(11), 712–719. doi:10.1097/00005053-199011000-00007

Ferrari, A. J., Charlson, F. J., Norman, R. E., Patten, S. B., Freedman, G., Murray, C. J., Vos, T., & Whiteford, H. A. (2013). Burden of depressive disorders by country, sex, age, and year: Findings from the global burden of disease study 2010. *PLoS Medicine, 10*(11), e1001547. https://doi.org/10.1371/journal.pmed.1001547

First, M. B., Gaebel, W., Maj, M., Stein, D. J., Kogan, C. S., Saunders, J. B., Poznyak, V. B., Gureje, O., Lewis-Fernández, R., Maercker, A., Brewin, C. R., Cloitre, M., Claudino, A., Pike, K. M., Baird, G., Skuse, D., Krueger, R. B., Briken, P., Burke, J. D., Lochman, J. E., ... Reed, G. M. (2021). An organization- and category-level comparison of diagnostic requirements for mental disorders in ICD-11 and DSM-5. *World Psychiatry, Official Journal of the World Psychiatric Association (WPA), 20*(1), 34–51. https://doi.org/10.1002/wps.20825

Government of Canada. (2019). *Suicide in Canada: Key statistics.* www.canada.ca/en/public-health/services/publications/healthy-living/suicidecanada-key-statistics-infographic.html

Grant, B. F., Goldstein, R. B., Saha, T. D., Chou, S. P., Jung, J., Zhang, H., Pickering, R. P., Ruan, W. J., Smith, S. M., Huang, B., & Hasin, D. S. (2015). Epidemiology of DSM-5 alcohol use disorder: Results from the National Epidemiologic Survey on alcohol and related conditions III. *JAMA Psychiatry, 72*(8), 757–766. doi:10.1001/jamapsychiatry.2015.0584

Hedden, S. L., Kennet, J., Lipari, R., Medley, G., Tice, P., Copello, E. A., & Kroutil, L. A. (2016). *Key substance use and mental health indicators in the United States: Results from the 2015 National Survey on Drug Use and Health.* Department of Health and Human Services.

Hudson, A., Thompson, K., MacNevin, P. D., Ivany, M., Teehan, M., Stuart, H., & Stewart, S. H. (2018). University students' perceptions of links between substance use and mental health: A qualitative focus group study. *Emerging Adulthood, 6*(6), 399–410.

Kann, L., Olsen, E. O. M., McManus, T., Harris, W. A., Shanklin, S. L., Flint, K. H., . . . Zaza, S. (2016). Sexual identity, sex of sexual contacts, and health-related behaviors among students in grades 9–12 – United States and selected sites, 2015. *Morbidity and Mortality Weekly Report: Surveillance Summaries, 65*(9), 1–202.

Kates, N., Mazowita, G., Lemire, F., Jayabarathan, A., Bland, R., Selby, P., . . . Audet, D. (2011). The evolution of collaborative mental health care in Canada: A shared vision for the future. *Canadian Journal of Psychiatry, 56*(5).

Khantzian, E. J. (1985). The self-medication hypothesis of addictive disorders: Focus on heroin and cocaine dependence. *American Journal of Psychiatry, 142*, 1259–1264. https://doi.org/10.1176/ajp.142.11.1259

Link, B. G., & Phelan, J. C. (2001). Conceptualizing stigma. *Annual Review of Sociology, 27*(1), 363–385.

Mereish, E. H., O'Cleirigh, C., & Bradford, J. B. (2014). Interrelationships between LGBT based victimization, suicide, and substance use problems in a diverse sample of sexual and gender minorities. *Psychology, Health & Medicine, 19*(1), 1–13.

Naghavi, M. (2019). Global, regional, and national burden of suicide mortality 1990 to 2016: Systematic analysis for the Global Burden of Disease Study 2016. *BMJ, 364*, 1–13. doi:10.1136/bmj.194

Patton, G. C., Coffey, C., Carlin, J. B., Degenhardt, L., Lynskey, M., & Hall, W. (2002). Cannabis use and mental health in young people: Cohort study. *British Medical Journal, 325*, 1195–1198. https://doi.org/10.1136/bmj.325.7374.1195

Public Health Agency of Canada, Centre for Chronic Disease Prevention. (2017). *The positive mental health surveillance indicator framework.* https://infobase.phacaspc.gc.ca/positive-mental-health

Reisner, S. L., Vetters, R., Leclerc, M., Zaslow, S., Wolfrum, S., Shumer, D., & Mimiaga, M. J. (2015). Mental health of transgender youth in care at an adolescent urban community health center: A matched retrospective cohort study. *Journal of Adolescent Health, 56*(3), 274–279.

Sheikh, S., & Furnham, A. (2000). A cross-cultural study of mental health beliefs and attitudes towards seeking professional help. *Social Psychiatry and Psychiatric Epidemiology, 35*, 326–334.

Statistics Canada. (2017). *Suicide rates: An overview.* https://www150.statcan.gc.ca/n1/pub/82-624-x/2012001/article/11696-eng.htm

Stewart, S. H., & Conrod, P. J. (Eds.). (2007). *Anxiety and substance use disorders: The vicious cycle of comorbidity.* Springer Science & Business Media.

Stewart, S. H., Grant, V. V., Mackie, C. J., & Conrod, P. J. (2016). Comorbidity of anxiety and depression with substance use disorders. In K. J. Sher (Ed.), *The Oxford handbook of substance use disorders* (Vol. 2). Oxford University Press. https://doi.org/10.1093/oxfordhb/9780199381708.001.0001

Tibbo, P., Crocker, C. E., Lam, R. W., Meyer, J., Sareen, J., & Aitchison, K. J. (2018). Implications of Cannabis legalization on youth and young adults. *Canadian Journal of Psychiatry, 63*, 65–71.

Williams, M. T., Printz, D., & DeLapp, R. C. (2018). Assessing racial trauma with the Trauma symptoms of discrimination scale. *Psychology of Violence, 8*(6), 735–749.

World Health Organization. (2015). *Premature death among people with severe mental disorders.* www.who.int/mental_health/management/info_sheet.pdf

CHAPTER 10

On the Importance of Aging and Health

10.0 Introduction

Now is a time for healthy aging! Or so said the United Nations on December 14, 2020,[1] when the United Nations General Assembly declared 2021 to 2030 the **decade of healthy aging.**

So how will we define healthy aging?

To begin, let's consider the hypothesis of Hanson and colleagues (2016), in which the authors suggested that the process of aging begins in conception and ends at death. For some, this process can be measured in minutes, while for others, it can extend more than 100 years. Clearly, this is a life course approach, with implicit limitations for specific events at milestone moments in the process of human development that can have significant impacts on the ability to achieve healthy aging. Of note here is the term *life course*, which Alwin (2012) described, and which is interpreted here as an integration of perspectives that describe the events – "causes and consequences" – that affect an individual and their development across their life cycle.

The challenge is, then, to define what we mean by healthy aging.

In a comprehensive review of the notion of healthy aging by Sadana and Michel (2019), the authors reported that for the year 2016, there were more than 3,000 new peer-reviewed papers published on the topic of healthy aging and an additional 500 papers published on the topic of successful aging. Given the plethora of information, identifying a common definition and road map to achieve healthy aging should be easy, but as the WHO indicated in the March 2019 introduction to the *decade of aging* and later in the 2022 follow-up report on aging,[2] there is no typical older person, and to achieve healthy aging means that one continues to develop and to maintain functional abilities that enable well-being throughout their life. Inherently, this approach supports the life course model of healthy aging and does not assume a single factor can be held responsible for success or failure in the pursuit of healthy aging (Menassa et al., 2023).

Rather, as Menassa and coworkers showed, the concepts of healthy aging can be sorted according to: (i) antecedents, which consist of both intrinsic and extrinsic factors

DOI: 10.4324/9781003474777-10

that act as precursors to outcomes; (ii) attributes, which include dimensions of development, such as physical, psychological, cognitive, environmental, political, economic, cultural, social, and spiritual dimensions, each of which has the potential to be interactive with the others and occurs throughout the life course; and (iii) consequences, which can be categorized as either subjective or objective and which can represent patterns of behavior within the aging process.

Mapping these three concepts together (antecedents, attributes, and consequences), we can create a rich matrix of explanations for healthy aging, and more importantly we can create a variety of different road maps to successfully achieve a life course model for healthy aging. Consider, for example, the intrinsic characteristics of the social demographics that a child is born into and combine them with considerations of the extrinsic factors of the built environment versus the natural environment. We know how valuable safety, security, and nurturing support are to maintain the physical, social, and psychological dimensions of health, and we have certainly seen the results of epigenetic studies that support the importance of these characteristics on disease development across the lifespan.

In the work of Menassa and colleagues, the authors summarized the combination of antecedents, attributes, and consequences into three basic types of healthy aging. In the first process model for healthy aging, the researchers suggest that healthy aging results from the interaction of both intrinsic (individual) and extrinsic (environmental) factors that lead to positive growth and development over the lifespan. In a second process model for healthy aging, the researchers suggest that healthy aging results from a dynamic method of adapting the characteristics of the antecedents and attributes to encourage positive interactions that prevent negative consequences. In this second type of aging, the healthy element is manifested through reliance on available support systems, which can include sociodemographic factors.

Finally, in a third process model for healthy aging, the researchers suggest that healthy aging results from a combination of characteristics from the first process model approach with those of the second process model approach to build resilience and empowerment and establish positive self-efficacy by pursuing goal-oriented behaviors. While these three approaches showed considerable overlap and consistency in characteristics, they are limited to the cohorts that contributed to the different research studies and the resulting literature that was used to organize the various models. Regardless, these models represent a comprehensive overview of considerations for healthy aging based on a positive approach to one's life course journey.

10.1 Ageism Is Nasty

Although there are models throughout the academic literature which describe positive practices to achieve healthy aging, not all aging is healthy, and not all aging is positive. Ageism, which Ayalon and Tesch-Römer (2017) defined as "stereotypes, prejudice, or discrimination against (but also in favour of) people because of their chronological age," is a ubiquitous negative practice across our global community. Although the practice can affect young persons, the most noted effects and ageist behaviors are researched and reported with reference to the cohort of individuals over 65 years of age – the cohort that we call older persons. Among the growing negative notions of aging that ultimately shape the attitude of ageism are the perspectives that older persons are merely the passive recipients of welfare, are an increasing burden to younger persons, and have little to no contributory value for society (Kang and Kim, 2022).

To identify explanatory factors for ageism against older people, Marques et al. (2020) conducted an extensive review of several research studies, and among the reported findings was that one of the key determinants of ageism was anxiety about aging among younger individuals. This finding was also reported in earlier work by Donizzetti (2019), who explained that anxiety about aging was manifested by a fear among younger persons because they didn't know how the aging process would affect them.

Donizzetti's work sought to evaluate the relationships between knowledge about aging, chronological age, stereotypes about the elderly, anxiety about aging, and ageism. Using a convenience sample of 886 participants with a 2-to-1 ratio of females to males, Donizzetti collected data on both cognitive and affective (i.e., emotional) aspects of ageism, along with measures of attitudes about older persons, overall anxiety about aging, and general knowledge about the aging process by presenting misconceptions of aging. While the observed outcomes lacked strong generalizability (APA, 2022), they supported the notion that increased knowledge about aging reduced the anxiety toward the aging process and led to positive attitudes toward aging, thereby demonstrating a potential to break the stereotypic perspectives of aging. As Donizzetti indicated, enhancing knowledge of aging is important to mitigating ageist behavior within younger cohorts. Ageism among younger persons does not reflect discrimination against a fixed cohort, like that which we might observe in prejudicial attitudes toward race, religion, or skin color. Rather, ageism – especially with respect to the younger-person-versus-older-person dynamic – points to the prejudice of one cohort (younger persons) toward another cohort (older persons), of which the younger cohort will become a member in the future.

Ageism results from societal values that lead to societal behaviors toward a particular cohort that is defined by chronological age. Once again, we restate that ageism is prejudice in its finest form. Ageism can be the prejudice that is directed toward younger persons, and ageism can be the prejudice that is directed to the cohort of older persons.

Ageism is a negative determining factor within the multiple elements that sustain an individual's health and well-being (Kang and Kim, 2022; Sabik, 2015). Throughout the aging process, individuals may feel a loss of self-worth, depression, anxiety, exclusion from society, and a loss of social value (Sabik, 2015). Ageism, which can be manifested through internalized self-perceptions or which can result from the external behaviors of others, exacerbates the adversities older persons experience during the aging process. As Sabik noted, previous research supports the idea that there is a direct positive association between "experiencing discrimination and poor psychological well-being (i.e., depression, psychological distress, anxiety, and well-being)" (Sabik, 2015, p. 192). Given that an individual's perception of others as well as their self-perception can be shaped by cultural values, Sabik (2015) hypothesized that ageist behaviors toward older women, along with negative values of aging women, could directly decrease psychological well-being among older women. To evaluate this hypothesis, Sabik (2015) examined the associations between perceptions of age discrimination, body esteem, health, and psychological well-being among late-middle-aged women. In conducting this research, Sabik surveyed some 244 women over 60 years of age to determine their perceptions of experiencing age discrimination, their body image, their subjective health, and overall feelings of well-being.

The results were not unexpected. That is, psychological well-being was positively associated with subjective health scores, which is interpreted as a rise in psychological well-being was directly associated with a rise in a respondent's perceived overall health. Likewise, poor psychological well-being reflected higher levels of age discrimination; and body image as determined by body esteem – the perception of feeling good about one's body image – was adversely affected by age discrimination but positively associated with psychological well-being. The latter finding means that as an individual's perception of their body esteem depreciated, so too did their psychological well-being.

The research by Sabik (2015) and later by Kang and Kim (2022) is noteworthy because it supports the contention that discrimination of any type has adverse effects on an individual's health and especially psychological well-being. Moreover, as we consider the effects of ageism and ageist behaviors on older persons, we can draw upon reliable and valid assessment tools that enable us to partition out the very specific causal effects of ageism on the health and psychological well-being of older persons. From this evidence, we can enrich health-promoting messages and shape health promotion programs that help to change the narrative about aging in a general sense, debunk the stereotypes that form the basis for implicit bias against older persons, and break the entrenched attitudes about chronological age determining worth and value of individuals in society.

10.2 Compression of Morbidity

Health promotion to establish a healthy aging trajectory would surely include behaviors that encourage if not ensure disease prevention among older persons. For some of us, as we continue our journey on our life cycle, we may find that prior to our death, we will experience a period of disability, when our existence is no longer under our own personal control. During this transition period from healthy aging to the end of our life, we may become dependent on support systems that ensure our existence. The duration of this disabled period near the end of life has enormous personal and societal implications. A disabled older adult has poorer quality of life and poorer health outcomes, including frequent hospital admissions and higher risk of mortality. Resultantly, the number of years lived under disability contributes greatly to overall healthcare costs. Informal caregiving, often by family members, also brings considerable yet less visible costs. Research indicates that the demands of caregiving place significant strain on caregivers, often contributing to mental health concerns such as depression and burnout as they try to balance caring for disabled older adult(s) with other family, work, and personal responsibilities (Schwarz and Roberts, 2000).

The compression of morbidity refers to the concept of squeezing or compressing the window of time between the onset of chronic illness or disability and the time at which a person dies. Dr. James Fries who formulated the compression of morbidity hypothesis as "by minimizing the number of years people suffer from chronic illness, we enable older people to live more successful, productive lives that benefit themselves and society" (p. 1163). His hypothesis stated that "if the age at the onset of the first chronic infirmity can be postponed more rapidly than the age of death, then the lifetime illness burden may be compressed into a shorter period of time nearer to the age of death" (p. 1163). Put simply, Fries theorized that healthy behaviors, practiced throughout one's life, could alter the health trajectory to include an extended period of good health until close to the end of life (Swartz, 2008).

At the time the hypothesis of compression of morbidity was published in 1980, an opposing view was held by many gerontologists and epidemiologists, namely that improvements in medicine and public health would prolong life, leading to more prevalent morbidity and chronic illness – a prediction coined the "failure of success" in 1977 by psychiatrist and epidemiologist Dr. Ernest Gruenberg. In order to refute this hypothesis and provide support for the compression-of-disease paradigm, research was required to prove that, together, lifestyle factors, health promotion, and preventative medicine lead to more drastic increases in the *health span*, or years of life lived without disability, than they do the *life span*, or total years of life.

A third position, falling somewhere between the failure of success and the compression of morbidity, was termed "dynamic equilibrium" by Dr. Kenneth Manton (1982), who anticipated that advancements in medical care would predict increased longevity and increased prevalence of disease but also reduced severity and disability from disease. The presence of conflicting views and a need for data to substantiate or dismiss them sparked a great deal of interest among the research community.

10.3 Proof of Concept

Central to Fries's work was an emphasis on health promotion and disease prevention, so we will consider relevant work in these areas that have provided partial evidence for the compression of morbidity hypothesis. Some of the earliest evidence comes from longitudinal research conducted through the Arthritis, Rheumatism, and Aging Medical Information System (ARAMIS) – a databank established by Fries himself and funded by the National Institute of Health (NIH). ARAMIS gave rise to two large longitudinal studies of aging aimed at testing the compression-of-morbidity hypothesis by investigating the effects of health promotion and prevention in delaying onset of disability. The first study followed almost 2,000 University of Pennsylvania alumni for 20 years to determine whether people with lower modifiable health risks had less cumulative disability. The findings from this study revealed that cumulative lifetime disability was four times greater in those who smoked, were obese, and did not exercise as compared to nonsmokers with healthy body weights who exercised. Further, the onset of disability was delayed by almost 8 years in the portion of the sample with the lowest health risk compared to the portion of the sample with the highest risk (Vita et al., 1998). A second study with ARAMIS was conducted with adults 50+ who were either members of a runners' club or community control participants. Over the course of the 13-year study, the runners developed disability at a rate of almost one-fourth of the control group and showed a postponement in disability by over 8 years relative to control participants (Wang et al., 2002). Together, the results of investigations of compression-of-morbidity models substantiate the recommendation that quality of life and, to an extent, quantity of life can be augmented by lifestyle factors implemented in earlier stages of life.

More recent research into the compression of the morbid period took place under the auspices of the U.S. Cardiovascular Health Study (CHS), a longitudinal cohort study of cardiovascular risk factors in adults aged 65+ (Jacob et al., 2016). A total of 5,888 eligible participants were recruited through Medicare beneficiaries in four U.S. communities and followed for 25 years as part of the study. While the average number of disabled years was approximately 2.9 for men and 4.5 for women, multiple lifestyle factors were associated with observed years of life (YoL), years of able life (YAL), and the percentage value for years of able life YAL/YoL%. Otherwise put, YoL can be thought of as the lifespan, YAL can be thought of as the health span or years of life in which one's health supports daily activities without difficulty, and YAL/YoL% can be conceived as the proportion of life lived in health, without disability.

To illustrate the compression of morbidity relative to years of quality life, consider a death that occurs at age 82, with 2 years of disability and 80 years of able life. Calculating the ratio of years of active living to years of life expressed as a percentage, we can show that a person who had 80 years of active living divided by 82 years of life and then multiplied by 100, the individual lived almost 98% of their life without any difficulty in fulfilling the activities of daily living.

Lifestyle factors that showed the greatest impact on the CHS study outcomes were distances walked, diet, body mass index, and smoking. More precisely, greater distances walked and higher-quality diet were associated with a relative compression of the disabled period, obesity was associated with a relative expansion of the disabled period, and smoking was associated with a loss of YoL and YAL, affecting both mortality and morbidity. These results support the contention that when given the right combination of lifestyle factors, the disabled period can be compressed to inflate the number of years lived free of disability.

10.4 The Burden of Chronic Disease

Aside from the occasional pandemic, which we now expect to experience every generation, in the developed world, we can consider that we are in an era where the major burdens of illness can be attributed to chronic disease. That is, in the developed world, which is primarily made up of the world's richest countries, the illnesses that societies will deal with are most likely to include heart disease, stroke, cancer, chronic obstructive pulmonary disease, and diabetes. As society ages well beyond the traditional age of retirement, which most governments set at 65 years, the proportion of individuals carrying the burden of chronic disease will increase (PHAC, 2020). As noted by government forecasting of population dynamics, this growing proportion of the total number of individuals with chronic disease will be within the cohort of older persons.

Earlier research that reported the results from the Framingham Heart Study revealed that at age 50, the lifetime risk for developing heart disease was 51.7% for men and 39.2% for women (Lloyd-Jones et al., 2002). Cardiovascular disease incidence appears to be declining somewhat, at least recently, but many researchers have noted that the prevalence of heart disease and stroke survivors has increased in the population (Lloyd-Jones et al., 2002; Greenlee et al., 2002). So while there has been a slight decrease in the risk of having a heart attack or stroke, there has been a corresponding increase in survivorship for both forms of cardiovascular disease. In fact, surveillance of mortality and morbidity trends in the U.S. suggests that compression of morbidity associated with cardiovascular disease has remained relatively stagnant over recent years.

Cancer is the second leading cause of mortality in North America after cardiovascular disease. Cancer is not a singular disease of different body tissues but, instead, a number of distinct diseases with different risk factors, treatments, and trends. Over the past three decades, we have seen significant decreases in mortality rates for various cancers, a trend associated with both reduced incidence rates and increases in survival due to more progressive treatments (Coleman et al., 2008). Decreases in lung cancer mortality are believed to be due to decreased incidence associated with reduced exposure to tobacco smoke. Reductions in mortality for other cancers – notably breast, colorectal, and prostate – are thought to reflect increased screening, earlier diagnosis, and therapeutic improvements. Together, these trends underline the importance of health behaviors, such as smoking cessation and participation in early screening programs. As an aside, the advances in screening also muddy our interpretation of trends in incidence rates documented in cancer registries, as these are affected by screening policies and programs. As with cardiovascular illness, the increase in survival from cancer, with comparatively minor reductions in incidence, has led to a higher prevalence of people living with this illness in the population.

Diabetes is also a major cause of mortality and morbidity in Canada and the U.S., with mortality rates for diabetics being about twice those of their age-matched peers. Numerous studies have reported increasing prevalence and incidence of diabetes in developed and developing countries (e.g., Crimmins, 2004). Trends in diabetes morbidity are thought to reflect growing rates of obesity in the population. Fortunately, advancements in diagnostic and prognostic biomarkers of the disease mean more precise prediction of disease progression and more targeted treatment.

What do trends in chronic disease tell us about the compression of morbidity?

Early in the 20th century, most of the increase in life expectancy was due to improvements in infant and childhood mortality. At present, recent increases in life expectancy are due to enhanced survival among the older adult population – the segment of the population most likely to carry the burden of chronic disease. Indeed, as we have seen in the earlier summary, the prevalence of major forms of chronic disease is on the rise. Yet given the latest medical developments, we tend to see reduced mortality and disability associated with chronic disease (Crimmins and Beltrán-Sánchez, 2011).

This increased prevalence of disease, with reduced occurrence of disability, could be argued to provide evidence for the dynamic-equilibrium paradigm proposed by Manton. However, we must acknowledge that compression of morbidity may be more or less visible in certain segments of the population. For instance, people with higher socioeconomic status, those with higher educational attainment, and those who engage in aerobic activity are all known to have significantly better long-term health outcomes, which may speak to a compression of disease among such individuals (Vita et al., 1998). As such, the compression of morbidity may be more apparent at the level of the individual or within specified subpopulations than in the population at large. Indeed, although smoking rates have decreased in the general population, many lifestyle factors, such as obesity and physical activity rates, have remained unchanged or have worsened over past decades, offsetting the disease compression that would be anticipated to accompany advancements in health promotion and healthcare.

We must also contend with the different constructs used to indicate morbidity and compression thereof, which can significantly affect our interpretations. For instance, disease is distinct from disability, and disability exists along a spectrum and is reflective of both the individual (i.e., whether the person has the ability to independently fulfill daily functions) and the environment (i.e., whether accommodations exist; whether barriers are present). We must make these necessary distinctions to more aptly capture not only whether morbidity exists but the meaning of a particular diagnosis for the individual – and society. We must also recognize the relevance of extending years of able life, along with compressing the period of disability, as this brings with it increased productivity, contributions to society, and enhanced quality of life for the individual, their family, and their community.

10.5 Aging in Place and Social Isolation

A consistent predictor of quality of life for older people is the opportunity and capacity to age in place. *Aging in place* is a phrase commonly used in aging policy and research and is typically viewed in a positive light for its ability to promote independence, autonomy, continued participation in familiar routines, and ongoing connection to social networks in the older adult's community of residence (Frank, 2002). There are also health systems implications that drive the goal of supporting older adults to remain in their homes for as long as possible, namely the significant costs associated with institutional care (Wiles et al., 2012).

Despite the many benefits of aging in place, there are also potential risks for community-dwelling older adults. For instance, indicators of social isolation, such as living alone, having a small social network, infrequent participation in social activities, and feelings of loneliness, have all been associated with physical and mental health risks in seniors. Human beings are social by nature, and high-quality social relationships are vital for health and well-being. More precisely, social activity has been associated with reduced risk for cardiovascular disease, cancers, osteoporosis, rheumatoid arthritis, and mortality. From a mental health perspective, social engagement has been found to lower the occurrence of mental health issues, such as depression, and to slow the progression of memory loss and age-related cognitive decline (Saczynski et al., 2006). In fact, a number of studies have found that cognitive function and social engagement are interrelated and tend to decline together, suggesting that social engagement may be an important marker for resilience against or susceptibility to cognitive impairment. However, it is unclear whether socializing protects against cognitive decline, whether cognitive decline precipitates social withdrawal, or whether both mechanisms operate in tandem.

Social isolation (objective lack of social contact with others) and loneliness (the subjective feeling of being isolated) are significant but underappreciated public health risks.[3] Many documents support high prevalence rates of both social isolation and loneliness among older adults. Circumstances that interfere with the ability to seek social interactions can include grief related to the loss of a spouse or close friend, physical conditions affecting mobility, presence of chronic pain, hearing loss, financial changes in retirement, and decreased sense of security in a fast-paced, ever-changing world. Family members are not always nearby, and for many seniors, family visits are restricted to selected holidays. For seniors, socializing is often not easy, and thus they are at risk of becoming socially isolated.

Data from the National Health and Aging Trends Study found that 24% of community-dwelling older adults are considered socially isolated, and a 2018 survey by the American Association of Retired Persons (AARP) Foundation found that more than one-third (35%) of adults aged 45 and older self-report they are lonely. Additionally, a 2018 study by the Kaiser Family Foundation reported that 22% of adults in the United States say they "often or always feel lonely, feel that they lack companionship, feel left out, or feel isolated from others" (NAS, 2019, p. xi).

The prevalence of social isolation and loneliness in older adults, along with the associated health consequences, emphasizes a role for the healthcare sector in addressing the impacts of these experiences among this population. Key objectives for healthcare programs aimed at promoting social engagement among older adults include:

1 Developing a more robust evidence base for effective assessment, prevention, and intervention strategies for social isolation and loneliness;
2 Translating current research into healthcare practices in order to reduce the negative health impacts of social isolation and loneliness;
3 Improving awareness of the health and medical impacts of social isolation and loneliness across the healthcare workforce and among members of the public;
4 Strengthening ongoing education and training related to social isolation and loneliness in older adults for the healthcare workforce; and
5 Creating ties between the healthcare system and community-based networks and resources that address social isolation and loneliness in older adults.

10.6 Conclusion

As discussed in this chapter, lifestyle factors may compress or expand the duration of the disabled period, relatively independent of their effect on life expectancy. Fries's compression-of-morbidity theory has changed the way we think about aging, positioning the issue of aging at the heart of public health and stressing the role of lifestyle at various stages of development in predicting how we will function in the final chapters of our life.

A disabled older adult has poorer quality of life and poorer health outcomes, including frequent hospital admissions and higher risk of mortality. Moreover, years lived with disability contribute substantially to healthcare costs, which are already projected to increase because of the aging of the baby boom generation. Prevention of disease through promotion of healthy lifestyle factors can reduce the public health burden due to disability as more adults reach old age.

Some have taken epidemiological trends in chronic diseases as evidence against the compression-of-morbidity hypothesis, suggesting that we are seeing increases in the occurrence of chronic illness as the population of older adults continues to grow. Yet cohort studies have reliably found that morbidity and disability are delayed in people with the lowest modifiable health risks and greatest preventative factors, lending weight to the notion that we can strategically shrink periods of ill health and disability and extend the number of years of productivity and good health.

There was a time when the health sciences community and the population at large commonly considered "healthy aging" to be an oxymoron, where the very process of aging was assumed to bring with it frailty and morbidity. However, progress in the field of gerontology has proven that lifestyle factors, largely under our control, have the potential to compress the disabled period toward the end of life, significantly extending the number of years characterized by health, ability, and self-sufficiency.

Finally, epidemiological data and research evidence support the conjecture that we can achieve healthy aging across society. However, the stigma of aging as a negative trajectory in an individual's life continues to plague social structures, and as such society, must be vigilant to address ageism as a blatant form of negative, prejudicial behavior that adversely affects psychological well-being.

10.6.1 Discussion Questions

1   Consider how the compression of morbidity can help the healthcare system. Discuss ways that we can use this information in the promotion of health and well-being to reduce the economic burden of infirmity related to morbidity.

2   What is meant by aging in place? Is the notion of aging in place a construct that society can promote with economic efficiency, or, ultimately, will it add to the economic burdens of society, not to mention the stress and strain on family and community supports?

Notes

1 www.who.int/docs/default-source/documents/decade-of-health-ageing/decade-healthy-ageing-update-march-2019.pdf?sfvrsn=5a6d0e5c_2
2 October 1, 2022 – Ageing and health (who.int).
3 Social isolation and loneliness represent distinct phenomena and are often uncorrelated. An individual can be isolated but not feel lonely or can be lonely even if they are not isolated. So it is important to distinguish between the two states.

References

Alwin, D. F. (2012). Integrating varieties of life course concepts. *Journals of Gerontology Series B: Psychological Sciences and Social Sciences, 67*(2), 206–220. doi:10.1093/geronb/gbr146

American Psychological Association (APA) (2022). https://dictionary.apa.org/generalizability

Ayalon, L., & Tesch-Römer, C. (2017). Taking a closer look at ageism: Self- and other-directed ageist attitudes and discrimination. *European Journal of Ageing, 14*(1), 1–4. doi:10.1007/s10433-016-0409-9

Coleman, M. P., Quaresma, M., Berrino, F., Lutz, J. M., De Angelis, R., Capocaccia, R., . . . CONCORD Working Group. (2008). Cancer survival in five continents: A worldwide population-based study (CONCORD). *The Lancet Oncology, 9*(8), 730–756.

Crimmins, E. M. (2004). Trends in the health of the elderly. *Annual Review of Public Health, 25*, 79–98.

Crimmins, E. M., & Beltrán-Sánchez, H. (2011). Mortality and morbidity trends: Is there compression of morbidity? *The Journals of Gerontology: Series B, 66*(1), 75–86.

Donizzetti, A. R. (2019). Ageism in an aging society: The role of knowledge, anxiety about aging, and stereotypes in young people and adults. *International Journal of Environmental Research and Public Health, 16*(8), 1329. doi:10.3390/ijerp6081329

Frank, J. B. (2002). *The paradox of aging in place in assisted living.* Greenwood Publishing Group.

Greenlee, R. T., Naleway, A. L., & Vidaillet, H. (2002). Incidence of myocardial infarction in a general population: The Marshfield Epidemiologic Study Area. *WMJ: Official Publication of the State Medical Society of Wisconsin, 101*(7), 46–52.

Hanson, M. A., Cooper, C., Aihie Sayer, A., Eendebak, R. J., Clough, G. F., & Beard, J. R. (2016). Developmental aspects of a life course approach to healthy aging. *Journal of Physiology, 594*, 2147–2160. doi:10.1113/JP270579

Jacob, M. E., Yee, L. M., Diehr, P. H., Arnold, A. M., Thielke, S. M., Chaves, P. H., . . . Newman, A. B. (2016). Can a healthy lifestyle compress the disabled period in older adults? *Journal of the American Geriatrics Society, 64*(10), 1952–1961.

Kang, H., & Kim, H. (2022). Ageism and psychological well-being among older adults: A systematic review. *Gerontology and Geriatric Medicine, 8.* doi:10.1177/23337214221087023

Lloyd-Jones, D. M., Larson, M. G., Leip, E. P., Beiser, A., D'Agostino, R. B., Kannel, W. B., . . . Levy, D. (2002). Lifetime risk for developing congestive heart failure: The Framingham Heart Study. *Circulation, 106*(24), 3068–3072.

Manton, K. G. (1982). Changing concepts of morbidity and mortality in the elderly population. *The Milbank Memorial Fund Quarterly Health and Society, 60*, 183–244.

Marques, S., Mariano, J., Mendonça, J., De Tavernier, W., Hess, M., Naegele, L. . . . Martins, D. (2020). Determinants of ageism against older adults: A systematic review. *International Journal of Environmental Research and Public Health, 17*(7), 2560. doi:10.3390/ijerp7072560

Menassa, M., Stronks, K., Khatmi, F., Roa Díaz, Z. M., Espinola, O. P., Gamba, M., . . . Franco, O. H. (2023). Concepts and definitions of healthy aging: A systematic review and synthesis of theoretical models. *EClinicalMedicine, 56*, 101821. doi:10.1016/j.eclinm.2022.101821

National Academies of Sciences (NAS), Engineering, and Medicine. (2019). *Reproducibility and replicability in science.* The National Academies Press. doi:10.17226/25303

PHAC: Public Health Agency of Canada. (2020). *Aging and chronic diseases: A profile of Canadian seniors (Cat.: HP35-137/1-2020E-PDF, Pub.: 200117).* http://canadian-seniors-report_2021-eng.pdf (canada.ca)

Sabik, N. J. (2015). Ageism and body esteem: Associations with psychological well-being among late middle-aged African American and European American women. *Journals of Gerontology Series B: Psychological Sciences and Social Sciences, 70*(2), 191–201. doi:10.1093/geronb/gbt080

Saczynski, J. S., Pfeifer, L. A., Masaki, K., Korf, E. S., Laurin, D., White, L., & Launer, L. J. (2006). The effect of social engagement on incident dementia: The Honolulu-Asia Aging Study. *American Journal of Epidemiology, 163*(5), 433–440.

Sadana, R., & Michel, J. P. (2019). Healthy aging: What is it and how to describe it? In J. P. Michel (Eds.), *Prevention of chronic diseases and age-related disability. Practical issues in geriatrics.* Springer. https://doi.org/10.1007/978-3-319-96529-1_2

Schwarz, K. A., & Roberts, B. L. (2000). Social support and strain of family caregivers of older adults. *Holistic Nursing Practice, 14*(2), 77–90.

Swartz, A. (2008). James Fries: Healthy aging pioneer. *American Journal of Public Health, 98*(7), 1163–1166.

Vita, A. J., Terry, R. B., Hubert, H. B., & Fries, J. F. (1998). Aging, health risks, and cumulative disability. *New England Journal of Medicine, 338*(15), 1035–1041.

Wang, B. W., Ramey, D. R., Schettler, J. D., Hubert, H. B., & Fries, J. F. (2002). Postponed development of disability in elderly runners: A 13-year longitudinal study. *Archives of Internal Medicine, 162*(20), 2285–2294.

Wiles, J. L., Leibing, A., Guberman, N., Reeve, J., & Allen, R. E. (2012). The meaning of "aging in place" to older people. *The Gerontologist, 52*(3), 357–366.

CHAPTER 11

Issues in Global Health

11.0 Introduction

To understand global health and, more importantly, to establish the impetus to effect positive change as health researchers, practitioners, clinicians, educators, promoters, and policymakers, we need to work from a definition that provides direction and appropriate functionality. In one of the most comprehensive definitions of global health, Koplan et al. (2009) combined the elements of public health with the qualities of international health to characterize the features of global health. Their definition for global health emerges from the public health concepts of evidence-based decision-making, consideration for a whole population approach, and establishing upstream prevention practices that extol the virtues of social justice and equity while drawing on the discipline of international health to recognize the importance of the dynamics of infectious diseases and the plight of individuals in low- and middle-income countries.

In creating their definition, Koplan and coworkers suggested that global health transcends boundaries, demands global cooperation, and addresses whole health at both the individual and population levels. Likewise, the concept of global health strives to achieve health equity among all nations by drawing on interdisciplinary and multidisciplinary practices that extend beyond the health sciences. Through this approach, Koplan and colleagues, who together represent the Executive Board of the Consortium of Universities for Global Health, contrasted and compared the utilities associated with global health, public health, and international health by illustrating the importance of geographical reach, levels of cooperation, population targets, access to health(care), and the range of disciplines that contribute to the three categories (global, international, and public health).

Global health is hard to define because it is truly complex, and with multiple meanings, it has earned the distinction that it is polysemous. However, in global health, the problems are more than merely complicated (Salm et al., 2021). Issues that arise as global health problems can be described as wicked problems because the resolutions require coordinated and cooperative transactions between individuals on a global scale. These transactions are rarely universally consistent with the central strategic missions and values of all collaborative partners and thus add to the complexity in establishing resolutions. Without question, global health issues require cooperation among stakeholders and decision-makers.

Building on the multiple definitions of global health presented by various authors (Salm et al., 2021), we can accept that global is not necessarily a place but is rather a scope. That is, the problems that one addresses in global health are broad and can influence populations on a global level regardless of race, ethnicity, political borders, and geographical constraints. We can also accept that global health is not limited to the low- and middle-income countries that are ravaged by military conflict, pestilence, and environmental calamities. Moreover, we can resolve that the issues of global health which are shown in various locations beyond our borders are also relevant in our local communities and thereby enable us to contribute to prevention if not solutions for the underlying causal mechanisms. In this way, we can consider that global health refers to the scope of the problem, being global in nature and not isolated to assisting only those individuals that exist in remote lands where most of us will never travel.

Global health need not be defined or described within a strictly medicalized context, as in the pursuit of approaches to eradicate a virus through the rapid development and deployment of a new vaccine. Similarly, global health should not be restricted to providing one-time mission support for refugees from a random natural disaster. Rather, in establishing a comprehensive understanding of global health, we continue to press that the term *global* refers to scope not place. Therefore, we can observe how issues like climate change that led to excessive monsoon related flooding in Islamabad, Pakistan, is absolutely related to the atmospheric rivers that caused flooding in Santa Barbara, California.

When we think of global as scope, we more readily understand that issues of global health are not restricted to locales that have definitive borders but that issues like food insecurity in parts of Europe and North America are a function of acts of aggression like Putin's illegal assault of Ukraine and the destabilization of food production and food distribution on a global scale. Correspondingly, viewing global health issues in this way exemplifies the need for cooperation amongst countries and the importance of developing strategies which privileged countries can follow, regardless of political differences, to resolve the issues, which in the case of food insecurity leads to restocking the storehouses of the world.

Accepting that global health is complex is important, especially if we begin to consider that the specific issues of global health can be addressed using non-traditional methodologies of problem-solving. For example, as noted by Faerron Guzmán (2022), adopting a complexity theory approach to resolving the wickedness of global health issues enables individuals to consider addressing problems beyond linear solutions and incorporating trans-disciplinary approaches that encourage cross-disciplinary sharing of information and knowledge. In a complexity theory application to address global health issues, we do not need to consider geo-political borders but rather to think of addressing the issues as part of a system that flows back and forth between global and local impacts. Addressing the wickedness of global health issues can build on our collective intelligence (Woolley et al., 2015; Williams, 2023) and bring together humans applying the tools of artificial intelligence to deal with the relevant issues by developing strategies that optimize possible interventions which will have the greatest impact on clearly defined problems. There is a general expectation that earlier research on the effectiveness of collective intelligence combined with the emergence of artificial intelligence as a contributor to heuristics that focus on health issues at a global level will at least contribute to new approaches to resolving old, wicked problems.

11.1 Considering Developmental Goals as a Road Map for Global Health Issues

We humans love to set goals.

In fact, we often set goals that are far-reaching, and for many of us, there is little chance that we will ever be successful in achieving such goals. As noted by Locke and Latham (2019) many organizations set goals as part of their reason for existence and as a target for organizational success. Consider the eight Millennial Development Goals that were established as part of the Millennial Declaration to which 189 countries signed on, in 2000 (Way, 2015).[1] Despite the fact that these goals were proposed at the start of this century we accept that they were simply goals, targets, or intentions, and their purpose was to provide direction and motivation toward a target. These Millennial Development Goals (2000–2015) were the precursor to the currently running Sustainable Development Goals of 2015–2030, and in both circumstances, we accept that MDGs and SDGs are aspirational and may never be achieved. However, just as we set goals, we also establish objectives as milestones along the path to achieve our goals (Ogbeiwi, 2017). Thus, our objectives are measured, assessed, evaluated, and translated, and therefore, the specific objectives can help us determine our success in striving toward our goals, especially from a global health perspective.

The main aspiration of the development goals, be they MDGs or SDGs, is that they were set with an end point for success and with an expectation of what could be achieved by a given date. However, neither the MDGs nor the SDGs could be considered as following the guidance of SMART goals, where SMART goals represent pursuits that are specific, measurable, attainable, realistic, and time-bound (Ogbeiwi, 2017). For both the set of MDGs and SDGs, we know that they were not nor could not be achieved on a global scale within a fixed time and be sustained globally. Yet as noted, these goals were aspirational. More important are the objectives that were set to measure change, to demonstrate positive gains that were realistic and attainable during the goal-pursuit journey. Despite the far-reaching characteristics of the MDGs and SDGs, there is evidence that major gains were realized. That is, simply by suggesting these goals, countries around the world began the process of planning strategies, implementing interventions, and identifying important milestones, a priori, for each development goal.

In both the MDGs and the SDGs, there was a call to eradicate hunger and poverty. A lofty goal indeed but a valuable target for our global community to rally around and establish as many strategies as possible for the nations of the world to achieve. Given the ever-emerging challenges which include but are not limited to ongoing drought and crop failure as a result of climate change and poor land management, military conflicts leading to displacement of populations and degrading resources, and the emergence of autocracies that foment conflict among societies and reduce financial support to countries in need, it is easy to see how this far-reaching goal will never be completely realized. Yet before the worldwide pandemic brought on by COVID-19, the world saw a tremendous decline in poverty rates. As noted by the United Nations report "*Ending Poverty | United Nations*,"[2] between 1990 and 2014 the percentage of persons living in poverty dropped from 37.8% to 11.2%, which reflected a 1.1% decline each year. However, this rate of poverty decrease began to slow as of 2014 and was drastically reduced because of the pandemic from 2020 to 2022. As of 2023, an estimated 10% of the world's population endured extreme poverty. An estimate which indicates that more than 700 million people exist on a daily income of less than USD$1.90 per day (*Poverty | UN Global Compact*[3]).

11.2 Is the Eradication of Poverty a Goal Too Far?

The simplest answer is no, because there are solutions that can ensure people are provided opportunities to earn a living wage beyond less than a couple of dollars per day. There are pathways out of poverty that require re-education and creating opportunities to learn new skills. There are opportunities for all members of society, regardless of gender, age, and ethnicity, to learn and earn a wage that is suitable for advancement in their social strata. However, this optimistic approach requires a global investment and a global acceptance of equity for all while halting our current pursuits in the developed world of individual advancement without consideration of those less fortunate. The solutions to success require that we recognize the potential negative health consequences of informal employment (Lee and Di Ruggiero, 2022) and the positive outcomes that can be achieved when equity, diversity, and inclusion are entrenched in the workplace globally (Chaudhry et al., 2021).

> *So what about a less contentious goal like achieving universal primary education?*

Of course, we think of achieving universal primary education as less contentious because it is such a simple concept. All we are asking is to establish the basics of literacy, numeracy, and the use of technology . . . for everyone!

According to Richards and Vining (2015), achieving this goal is not as easy as one might think, and it is even less obvious in low-income countries. The success or failure to achieve and sustain the goal of universal primary education depends on literacy levels of parents, the political will of local governments to support the enhancement and saturated distribution of primary education across the state, and especially the recognition and implementation of necessary investment in the essential capital to provide the resources for global education. These factors may seem inconsequential in a high-income country with a somewhat stable democracy, but as noted by Bamik (2018), in a country like Afghanistan, where Taliban rule controls the culture and the free movement of goods and services not only geographically but across the social fabric of society, education of half the population – aka females – is challenged by religious and cultural restrictions. As Bamik stated, the male domination of Afghanistan society restricts activities and the natural growth and human development of its citizenry, and especially for girls. In a country like Afghanistan, girls really are second class, and for the most part in the social hierarchy of a family are provided the leftovers after the male has had his choice. This includes the provision of education where Bamik indicated that education for girls is neither promoted nor encouraged.

Gender inequality isn't isolated to one country and to one religious belief. On both a local and a global scale, the pursuit of gender equality has several challenges which can be described in absolute terms as wicked problems. Establishing gender equality is the basis for our pursuit of Goal 5 of the SDGs; it is a fundamental tenet for the establishment of a healthy global population, and as noted by Weber et al. (2019), it is a basic human right. Yet gender equality, as a sustainable development goal, will not be achieved by the 2030 target date because much of the world continues to suffer from **gender-blindness.**

By stating explicitly the need to pursue gender equality as a goal for both the MDGs and the SDGs, we accept that gender equality does not exist, not locally in many realms and therefore not globally. In fact, the report of the United Nations Department of Economic and Social Affairs (2022)[4] stated that the world is 300 years away from achieving gender equity if we remain on our current path.

Research by Cislaghi et al. (2020) showed that there is a need to address the social intersections of health across both sex and gender in order for society to achieve greater health and well-being in a global health context. Moreover, the Series on Gender Equality, Norms, and Health published by *The Lancet* in 2019[5] provides comprehensive evidence that is necessary to increase the momentum in addressing gender inequities in the pursuit of positive health for society.

One way we can begin to address the gender inequities that exist in regard to health is to confront the gender norms that continue to shape the health and well-being outcomes of marginalized individuals, predominantly women and girls, across many global societies. The term *gender norms* refers to the socially constructed spoken and unspoken rules that shape behaviors, activities, access to resources, and as Weber and coworkers described, even how individuals within a society think and feel. Gender norms are inhibitors to achieving positive states of health and well-being, especially among women and girls, and members of the LGBTQIA2S+ communities, as well as cohorts of men and boys in specific communities. Gender norms are relevant as they shape our societies because they shape our expectations. In discussions of gender norms, we might quickly jump to the scenario of a male-dominated society in which religious or cultural beliefs restrict growth and development among girls and women, as we did here in our example of the country of Afghanistan and the controls of the Taliban. Similarly, we might be quick to point out how laws are enacted to prevent the free expression of sexual preference or non-binary identities, but in previous work by Weber and colleagues, the researchers showed how gender norms are truly a global health issue because they are present in all societies. That is, gender norms, by definition, are not sex specific but are socially constructed so that given the context, gender norms can have a direct effect on boys, men, and non-binary individuals as much as they can have a direct effect on girls and women.

Yet many of us are aware of stories from various societies in which girls have less value than boys (Heise et al., 2019) because the gender norms are fundamental to supporting a patriarchal society. As a result, we see the perpetuation of attitudes wherein a positive change toward gender equity can never happen because the predominant male culture is entrenched. For example, Tesha et al. (2023) described the situation in Tanzania in which women are restricted from access to many health services because they lack control over resources. Lacking gender equity within such societies perpetuates the imbalance of power and therefore inhibits the potential for economic gain which could lead to better resource allocation. Despite that males have greater access to economic advantages in these communities, such advantages do not necessarily constitute actual realization of holding financial resources. As Tesha and coworkers found, men in these communities reported that they struggle with poverty as a major challenge to fulfilling their role as the primary income earner for their families. In turn, these challenges have a knock-on effect on their female partners and family members and can restrict these individuals from having access to health services in general and reproductive services specifically.

However, just as there are stories of the negative consequences for health system access because of a predominant male culture, there are growing numbers of reports of positive outcomes for women and girls in communities where laws and, subsequently, cultural traditions are changing to break the cycle of predominant male bias (Gupta et al., 2019). As Gupta and coworkers indicated, researchers have shown that by engaging individuals across genders in programs that illustrate the inequities explicitly, the communities give voice to the situation and demonstrate how changing these gender norms can lead to positive outcomes. Research by Bapolisi et al. (2024), showed that in the Democratic Republic of the Congo, by sensitizing men to the issues of gender-norming behaviors and concomitantly enabling women to pursue economic development activities, the community could realize positive household economic prosperity and enhance access to health services while also reducing food insecurity. However, this move toward a paradigm shift in which the male, as the head of the household and thus the primary provider, was not without frustration within households nor without the tug-of-war that accompanies culture change. Had this been a simple, widely accepted panacea to the issues of gender inequity and non-traditional empowerment of women in a household, the results may have been more profound and demonstrated a greater positive effect.

11.3 Health Literacy and Global Health Issues

Health literacy is indeed a global health issue in and of itself, but how does health literacy or lack thereof influence global health issues? Earlier, in Chapter 5, we said that most often, definitions of health literacy emphasize an individual's ability to obtain, understand, appraise, and apply information that is specific to maintaining or enhancing one's health. From a global health perspective, we realize that suggesting a definition that is plausible is one thing, but operationalizing the definition may be quite difficult, especially given the constraints and limitations that face individuals across cultures and social demographic strata.

In July of 2023, the World Health Organization released its report entitled *Advancing the Global Agenda on Prevention and Control of Non-Communicable Diseases 2000 to 2020: Looking Forwards to 2030*. This WHO report describes the increased prevalence of deaths attributable to non-communicable diseases (NCD) as rising from 61% in 2000 to 74% in 2019 and how this trend is affecting individuals from age cohorts between 30 and 70 years of age, when humans are most productive and thus able to provide the greatest quality of life to themselves and their families. Moreover, as one could certainly predict, the greatest burden of premature deaths attributed to NCD occur in the low- to middle-income countries (LMIC).

Research by Osborne et al. (2022) points to health literacy or lack thereof as a major challenge for societies globally to deal with risk factors that lead to the slow but progressive development of non-communicable diseases. As a primary example, Osborne discusses the influence of profit-motivated companies that saturate the marketplace with misinformation about the virtues of products like alcohol, tobacco, and sugary drinks without regard for the physical health consequences of continuous consumption of these products. It takes decades to develop a really good case of a non-communicable disease like coronary heart disease, so most individuals fail to regard the risk factors that cause the disease as well as the warning signs that their NCD is progressing. Moreover, the outcome of NCDs is not merely physical degradation but, as noted by Osborne and the WHO, NCDs are linked to genetic, physiological, environmental, and behavioral risk factors.

Given that NCDs are predominantly in low- to middle-income countries, where poverty is also prominent, it is expected that the association between NCDs and poverty is strong, and the inability to move the needle on poverty reduction is a function of the ever-growing burden of NCD prevalence. NCD prevalence is a wicked health problem in that the complexity of NCD prevalence both locally and globally has tremendous potential for social upheaval. As individuals continue to ignore the necessary steps to mitigate the modifiable risk factors for NCD, such as avoiding tobacco use, physical inactivity, substance use – especially excessive alcohol consumption – and adopting an unhealthy diet, the social and financial burden of disease treatment and eventual quality of life years lost can be severely detrimental to communities, with both local and global implications.

Osborne and coworkers (2022) suggested an approach to enhancing health literacy within a community using a strategy that is based on five action items which they deemed to be *appropriate, meaningful, and useful in different community and country contexts*. The authors suggested that adopting such a strategy can help to reduce the misinformation associated with lifestyle and modifiable risk factors and, instead, enhance an individual's ability to deal with risk factors that lead to NCDs. In particular, the strategy builds on existing successful intervention approaches within communities, increases access to accurate, relevant, and actionable information for citizens to increase opportunities for health literacy development among members of the community, continues to develop the health literacy of the health workforce, and strengthens the competencies and trust of the leaders in the community. This approach is not geographically specific but maintains the necessary universal application that can enable application of such a strategy in any community. Developing a learning system within the community that recognizes the need to enhance literacy across these criteria will be relevant globally and will contribute to the mitigation of negative information that predisposes individuals to the risk factors for NCDs.

11.4 Child Mortality Is a Global Health Issue

Finally, a conversation on global health would not be complete without raising issues of childhood mortality and how we can help to reduce childhood mortality globally. Improved access to nutritious foods, clean water, and vaccines – especially during early childhood development – are each major positive factors that help to reduce childhood mortality. Add to these factors enhanced neonatal healthcare, improved sanitation, and increased access to appropriate and affordable medicines, and we can explain the noticeable decline in childhood mortality – especially in the LMICs of the developing world. But as Cheng and Shilkofski (2019) suggest, our goals should evolve from helping children survive to ensuring that children thrive. As noted, far too many children are growing up in a world of distress in which their hope is not for glorious opportunities as they grow into young adults. Rather, their hope is to merely exist, to find secure shelter, a safe community without the threat of imminent death, and nourishment of any kind daily. Imagine waking each day and wondering if today is your last, like yesterday was for your friends or members of your immediate family. Children are not the decision-makers in the world that decide where, and when to drop bombs, rape and torture innocent victims, or steal valuable commodities that can provide quality to the lives of so many. But children are the nameless victims that die or suffer through the pain and hardship imposed by thoughtless megalomaniacs, terrorists, and leaders that are so consumed by greed for power and control that they perpetuate man's inhumanity to man.

The health of a country is evaluated on several indices, many of which have future financial growth and success indicators as underlying tenets. Among these indices is the future life years lost because of premature death among members of the population. The premature death of children is important to these indices because life lost within this cohort represents a future void for the country's population and thus a decrease in future life years – of potential productivity within the population. As a global community, we continue to address the issues of child mortality by setting goals for mortality rates relative to age. In addition to the infant mortality rate – the number of deaths among newborns, which is expressed as the number of infant deaths per 1,000 live births (Gonzalez and Gilleskie, 2017) – we also report the child mortality rate. The child mortality rate is based on the number of children who die before they reach the age of 5 years – a term we refer to as the under 5 mortality rate (U5MR) (Guillot et al., 2012). As noted by Guillot and colleagues, as part of the year 2000 MDGs, the United Nations pledged to reduce the U5MR to less than one-third of the 1990 mortality rate by the year 2015. Although this was believed to be a reasonable target, there were many underlying factors that were not considered in establishing this goal. Notwithstanding the variance in estimates of mortality that are reported across countries because of data reporting errors, differences in epidemiology practices, and the inconsistencies in using a standardized estimation process for all countries (Gonzalez and Gilleskie, 2017; Guillot et al., 2012), there is also the random but regular occurrence of war, natural disasters, emerging infectious diseases, and migration that has both direct and indirect effects on our ability to establish accurate estimates of infant mortality rate (IMR) and the under 5 years of age mortality rate (U5MR). As reported by Madewell et al. (2022), by establishing a more accurate estimate of mortality rates among children and determining the likely causes of death within this cohort of the population, we can move forward to identify gaps and challenges in the social fabric of a society and target our energy to enhance the systems that not only prevent premature deaths but support the community to reduce the risk factors that lead to such early years of life lost.

11.5 Conclusion

There are no simple solutions to reduce the IMR or the U5MR as part of our intended contribution to enhancing global health. Drought and famine are very real, and these are the existential challenges many children and unborn fetuses face each day. As a community of like-minded health researchers, practitioners, clinicians, educators, promoters, and policymakers, we need to recognize these challenges and focus our energy on addressing the wicked problems that underlie global health issues. What this means is that the collective WE need to focus not on the immediate issues of the multiple calamities that disproportionately affect humanity but rather to address the underlying causes of such calamities. In our community of practice, we need to be forthright in our conviction to address the real causes of global health issues. These causes are not based on immediacy to treat illness, but rather these causes are social, financial, educational, political, and based in ignorance. These causes are the root of the climate crisis, the relentless pursuit of manufacturing of unnecessary goods in an overheated Anthropocene, the disregard of the value of every human, and the want to control geographical spaces. These causes are the root of the greed that is pervasive in our global community and misguided lifestyle pursuits that lead to unwieldy global health crises. To address the causes of global health issues is not to pursue the eradication of disease and infirmity; rather, to address the causes of global health issues is to recognize the true meaning of HEALTH and to realize that global health issues are a function of the social, political, and economic determinants of health (Holst, 2020).

11.5.1 Discussion Questions

1 Global health issues are part of the wickedness of health problems. Is it possible for us to contribute positively to resolving global health issues? If we can contribute positively to global health issues, provide strategies that can be used. If we cannot contribute positively to global health issues, provide reasons we are restricted from doing so.
2 Consider the United Nations Sustainable Development Goals. Will they ever be achieved? Does it make sense to continuously list such goals in this way, or should we refrain from establishing these goals and rather simply state objectives for existing programs?

Notes

1 The eight Millennial Goals were the precursor to the subsequent 17 Sustainable Development Goals accepted in 2015 by the United Nations General Assembly Open Working Group (OWG). From MDGs to SDGs | Sustainable Development Goals Fund (sdgfund.org).
2 www.un.org/en/global-issues/ending-poverty
3 https://unglobalcompact.org/what-is-gc/our-work/social/poverty
4 https://t.co/CEAUazTV9J#SDG5 – report of the UN-Dept of Economic and Social Affairs (2022).
5 Gender Equality, Norms, and Health (thelancet.com) Published Online May 30, 2019 http://dx.doi.org/10.1016/S0140-6736(19)30985-7

References

Bamik, H. (2018). Afghanistan's cultural norms and girls' education: Access and challenges. *International Journal for Innovative Research in Multidisciplinary Field*, 4(11).
Bapolisi, W. A., Makelele, J., Ferrari, G., Kono-Tange, L., Bisimwa, G., Schindler, C., & Merten, S. (2024). Engaging men in women's empowerment: Impact of a complex gender transformative intervention on household socio-economic and health outcomes in the eastern democratic republic of the Congo using a longitudinal survey. *BMC Public Health*, 24(1), 443. doi:10.1186/s12889-024-17717-5

Chaudhry, I. S., Paquibut, R. Y., Tunio, M. N., & Wright, L. T. (2021). Do workforce diversity, inclusion practices, & organizational characteristics contribute to organizational innovation? Evidence from the U.A.E. *Cogent Business & Management*, 8(1). doi:10.1080/23311975.2021.1947549

Chen, X., Li, H., Lucero-Prisno, D. E. 3rd, Abdullah, A. S., Huang, J., Laurence, C., Liang, X., Ma, Z., Mao, Z., Ren, R., Wu, S., Wang, N., Wang, P., Wang, T., Yan, H., & Zou, Y. (2020). What is global health? Key concepts and clarification of misperceptions: Report of the 2019 GHRP editorial meeting. *Global Health Research and Policy*, 5, 14. doi:10.1186/s41256-020-00142-7

Cheng, T. L., Shilkofski, N., & for the Pediatric Policy Council. (2019). Global child health: Beyond surviving to thriving. *Pediatric Research*, 86, 683–684. doi:10.1038/s41390-019-0574-6

Cislaghi, B., Weber, A. M., Gupta, G. R., & Darmstadt, G. L. (2020). Gender equality and global health: Intersecting political challenges. *Journal of Global Health*, 10(1), 010701. doi:10.7189/jogh.10.010701

Faerron Guzmán, C. A. (2022). Complexity in global health–bridging theory and practice. *Annals of Global Health*, 88(1), 49, 1–8. doi:10.5334/aogh.3758

Gonzalez, R. M., & Gilleskie, D. (2017). Infant mortality rate as a measure of a country's health: A robust method to improve reliability and comparability. *Demography*, 54(2), 701–720. doi:10.1007/s13524-017-0553-7

Guillot, M., Gerland, P., Pelletier, F., & Saabneh, A. (2012). Child mortality estimation: A global overview of infant and child mortality age patterns in light of new empirical data. *PLoS Medicine*, 9(8), e1001299. doi:10.1371/journal.pmed.1001299

Gupta, G. R., Oomman, N., Grown, C., Conn, K., Hawkes, S., Shawar, Y. R., Shiffman, J., Buse, K., Mehra, R., Bah, C. A., Heise, L., Greene, M. E., Weber, A. M., Heymann, J., Hay, K., Raj, A., Henry, S., Klugman, J., Darmstadt, G. L., & Gender Equality, Norms, and Health Steering Committee (2019). Gender equality and gender norms: Framing the opportunities for health. *Lancet*, 393(10190), 2550–2562. doi:10.1016/S0140-6736(19)30651-8

Heise, L., Greene, M. E., Opper, N., Stavropoulou, M., Harper, C., Nascimento, M., & Zewdie, D. (2019). Gender equality, norms, and health: Gender inequality and restrictive gender norms: Framing the challenges to health. *The Lancet*, 393, 2440–2454.

Holst, J. (2020). The world expects effective global health interventions: Can global health deliver? *Global Public Health*, 15(9), 1396–1403. doi:10.1080/17441692.2020.1795222.

Koplan, J. P., Bond, T. C., Merson, M. H., Reddy, K. S., Rodriguez, M. H., Sewankambo, N. K., Wasserheit, J. N., & Consortium of Universities for Global Health Executive Board. (2009). Towards a common definition of global health. *The Lancet*, 373(9679), 1993–1995. doi:10.1016/S0140-6736(09)60332-9

Lee, J., & Di Ruggiero, E. (2022). How does informal employment affect health and health equity? Emerging gaps in research from a scoping review and modified e-Delphi survey. *International Journal for Equity in Health*, 21, 87. doi:10.1186/s12939-022-01684-7

Locke, E. A., & Latham, G. P. (2019). The development of goal setting theory: A half century retrospective. *Motivation Science*, 5(2), 93–105. doi:10.1037/mot0000127

Madewell, Z. J., Whitney, C. G., Velaphi, S., Mutevedzi, P., Mahtab, S., Madhi, S. A., Fritz, A., Swaray-Deen, A., Sesay, T., Ogbuanu, I. U., Mannah, M. T., Xerinda, E. G., Sitoe, A., Mandomando, I., Bassat, Q., Ajanovic, S., Tapia, M. D., Sow, S. O., Mehta, A., Kotloff, K. L., … Child Health and Mortality Prevention Surveillance Network (2022). Prioritizing health care strategies to reduce childhood mortality. *JAMA Network Open.* 5(10), e2237689. doi:10.1001/jamanetworkopen.2022.37689

Ogbeiwi, O. (2017). Why written objectives need to be really SMART. *British Journal of Healthcare Management*, 23, 324–336. doi:10.12968/bjhc.2017.23.7.324

Osborne, R. H., Elmer, S., Hawkins, M., et al. (2022). Health literacy development is central to the prevention and control of non-communicable diseases. *BMJ Global Health*, 7(12), e010362. doi:10.1136/bmjgh-2022-010362

Richards, J., & Vining, A. R. (2015). Universal primary education in low-income countries: The contributing role of national governance. *International Journal of Educational Development*, *40*, 174–182. doi:10.1016/j.ijedudev.2014.09.004

Salm, M., Ali, M., Minihane, M., & Conrad, P. (2021). Defining global health: Findings from a systematic review and thematic analysis of the literature. *BMJ Global Health*, 6, e005292. doi:10.1136/bmjgh-2021–005292

Tesha, J., Fabian, A., Mkuwa, S., Misungwi, G., & Ngalesoni, F. (2023). The role of gender inequities in women's access to reproductive health services: A population-level study of Simiyu Region Tanzania. *BMC Public Health*, 23, 1111. doi:10.1186/s12889-023-15839-w

UN-Dept of Economic and Social Affairs. (2022). *Progress on the sustainable development goals: The gender snapshot 2022*. Retrieved from https://www.unwomen.org/en/digital-library/publications/2022/09/progress-on-the-sustainable-development-goals-the-gender-snapshot-2022 on 9 April 2024.

Way, C. (2015). *The millennium development goals report 2015: Learning from progress* (75 pages). United Nations. undp.org

Weber, A. M., Cislaghi, B., Meausoone, V., & Abdalla, S. (2019). Gender norms and health: Insights from global survey data. *The Lancet*, *393*(10189), 2455–2468.

Williams, A. E. (2023). Are wicked problems a lack of general collective intelligence? *AI & Society*, *38*, 343–348. doi:10.1007/s00146-021-01297-8

Woolley, A. W., Aggarwal, I., & Malone, T. W. (2015). Collective intelligence and group performance. *Current Directions in Psychological Science*, *24*(6), 420–424. doi:10.1177/0963721415599543

World Health Organization (WHO). (2023). *Advancing the global agenda on prevention and control of noncommunicable diseases 2000 to 2020: Looking forwards to 2030*. World Health Organization.

CHAPTER 12

Planetary Health in the Age of the Anthropocene

12.0 Introduction

Here, we discuss planetary health and how human activity has changed the planet, the constituents of the biosphere, and the health of humanity.

We live on planet Earth. This is a fixed environment that is protected from the external universe by five thin layers of gases and particulate matter, beginning at sea level and extending 400kilometers outward (UCAR, 2023). Labelled in ascending order from the *terra firma* (Latin phrase for dry land), the five layers of gases include the troposphere, the stratosphere, the mesosphere, the ionosphere, and the thermosphere – the final separation between Earth and outer space (*aka the exosphere*).

While each of these layers is essential to maintain the balance of life on Earth, the troposphere is the layer in which we live. We exist in the troposphere as part of the community of ecosystems known as the biosphere. The biosphere was defined by Folke et al. (2011) as "the global ecological system" that shares resources between all living entities. The biosphere denotes all of the flora and fauna on planet Earth.

The constituents of the biosphere are alive and influenced by the activities of humans. As humans, we need to recognize that we are sharing space in the biosphere with all living elements, and thus, our actions have consequences for both our existence and for the existence of all other members of the biosphere. As important as we are, we cannot disregard the non-living elements of planet Earth – the abiotic elements – which not only provide us with essential resources, but which are finite and fragile. Understanding the effects of human activity on both the biosphere and the non-living elements of our planet are important to maintaining planetary health and the health of our species.

12.1 The Anthropocene – the Age of Mankind

The age of the Earth is measured not in years but in reference to a geological time clock, which describes the existence of our planet using eons that can be divided into eras and in which exist periods or epochs. Steffan et al. (2007) suggested that we are currently in the midst of a new geological time period that we have labelled *the Anthropocene*. Considering Earth's geological time record beginning with the Paleozoic era and moving forward past the age of dinosaurs in the Mesozoic era and into the Cenozoic era, the Anthropocene represents the most recent epoch (i.e., measured time period) within the Cenozoic era. According to Steffan and colleagues, the period of the Anthropocene began around the mid-1800s with the introduction of the industrial revolution and has continued to the present day. The period of the Anthropocene is derived from the term *anthropo* – as in human – and *cene*, which is used in describing a period within an era of geologic time. Hence these researchers refer to the Anthropocene as the "age of mankind."

The Anthropocene is marked as a period of tremendous flux within the biosphere.

This era accounts for the migration of humans away from agrarian economies and subsistence farming to widescale production of commodities with little regard for the impact of such activities on the biosphere. Herein lies the wicked problem of human development and our shared responsibility to our co-constituents in the biosphere along with our interaction with the non-living elements of our planet.

The Anthropocene denotes the accelerated impact of the human quest for development across a broad spectrum of measurable outcomes, some of which led to positive advancements in our civilizations as well as in the advancement of the positive states of health of humans. For example, during the Anthropocene, we accomplished tremendous progress in the production of mechanisms to make our work and everyday life tasks easier. We created new strategies to genetically modify food so that we could increase product yield, reduce crop failure, and enhance nutrient composition. We improved travel on land, on sea, and in the air as well as into outer space. We built economies on the use of fuel sources that not only include fossil fuel resources but also include natural energy sources such as solar energy, wind, water, tidal flows, and nuclear.

In the life sciences, we discovered ways to reduce the risks of disease through illness prevention and health promotion, by recognizing the relationship between phenotypic information aligned with genomic data (Robinson, 2012), including various new and emerging treatments, strategies for harm reduction, and the use of widespread and regularly scheduled vaccination programs. We improved the quality of life through rehabilitation and the replacement of body parts that are either worn out or non-functional. These are but a few of the many accomplishments that have enhanced the quality of life for our current existence on Earth. However, much of what we have done has been without consideration of the collateral damage to the other constituents and natural elements in the biosphere. Increased concentrations of human populations, leading to increased urbanization and encroachment on natural habitats, tied with the associated effects of climate change, are among the direct causal mechanisms of negative impacts on the biosphere. Consequentially, such adverse impacts are leading to negative health for the entire species of *Homo sapiens* – that's us!

Emblematic of the Anthropocene age has been the impact of increased population density on the biosphere. The rapid growth of human populations and the uncontrolled infringement of these populations on the natural environment has led to an unprecedented mixing and removal of habitats and the subsequent reduction in biodiversity. As habitats give way to human development and species become extinct at rates that range from 100 to 1,000 times higher than that which occurred in the past 1 billion years (May, 2011), the normal flow of life in the biosphere is in peril. However, since many of us have not yet recognized the impacts of lost biodiversity or our reckless exploitation of the non-living elements of the planet, we do not view these events as part of the wicked problem of human development within the Anthropocene.

Yet loss of biodiversity is only one of the many calamities that we face as we continue to add pressure to our fragile biosphere. The COVID-19 pandemic became a real and present threat to our existence and our normal way of life. Was it because of our hubris that we ignored our infringement on the habitats of our neighbors in the biosphere, or was it because we had lulled ourselves into a false sense of superiority over the constituents of the biosphere? Perhaps the COVID-19 pandemic has awakened us to another threat that has become a hallmark of the Anthropocene and which again is linked to population density and our disrespect of our fellow constituents in the biosphere.

Recognizing that humans have disproportionately contributed to the devastation of planet Earth has produced a level of mental stress that is real and measurable (Cianconi et al., 2020). The extreme weather events that are directly related to climate change and which are a consequence of human activities during the Anthropocene are both directly and indirectly considered to be the cause of an increased prevalence of negative mental health symptoms reported by individuals. For example, Cianconi et al. (2020) observed that the typical reports of climate change–related health symptoms include but are not limited to symptoms of distress, anxiety, and depression along with sleep disturbances and suicidal ideation. While there remains considerable work to be done that can help identify contributing causal factors, researchers are gaining a better understanding of the complexity of negative mental health issues associated with extreme weather events. Findings from an eight-year longitudinal study of adolescents by Sciberras and Fernando (2022) found that individuals with a high persistence of worry, explicitly about climate change, were more likely to develop depressive symptoms in late adolescence compared to adolescents with low to moderate levels of worry about climate change. Moreover, the researchers attributed the source of worry to the greater awareness among individuals in the sample cohort to their societal engagement in the discourse of climate chaos across various forms of social media and news reports (Sciberras and Fernando, 2022).

12.2 Climate Change and Human Health

While climate change, which is defined as "a change in the pattern of weather, and related changes in oceans, land surfaces and ice sheets, occurring over time scales of decades or longer,"[1] by itself is a wicked problem (Ireland et al., 2012), the relationship between human health and climate change is extremely complex because it is disproportionately influenced and influential across the planet. The noted complexity between human health and climate change is dependent on a multiplicity of factors, including the physical and social determinants of health, that for the most part are ignored by the broader fabric of society. The effect of global warming and climate change on the physical and social determinants of health is not a new topic for scientists or government decision-makers. The former vice-president of the United States, Al Gore, described the rising heat waves in the U.S. as a consequence of climate change in 1993. Likewise, Dr. Margaret Chan (former director general of the WHO) stated in 2008, "The warming of the planet will be gradual, but the effects of extreme weather events – more storms, floods, droughts, and heatwaves – will be abrupt and acutely felt. Both trends can affect some of the most fundamental determinants of health: air, water, food, shelter, and freedom from disease."

Yet despite the gradual pace of climate change, the people most at risk from general apathy and ignorance to a rapidly changing global climate will be those who are most disadvantaged. Marginalized and poor populations – aka the intentionally ignored – will suffer more devastating effects of climate change, more often and at a greater cost to their health than those who are well situated in developed environments and who can afford to act sooner to mitigate potential effects. Food and water insecurity, leading to higher costs and shortages of essential commodities, will be among the early bellwether events, followed by loss of income and opportunities to maintain livelihood through work or government support. The consequences of climate change on place – as in loss of land through coastal erosion, wildfires, floods, and landslides – will lead to population displacement and, in some instances, forced migration.

Pakistan is a country that has seen tremendous devastation as a result of climate change in more recent times. Severe heat waves during the spring months of March to May 2022, in which the average daily temperature rose above 50° Celsius, were followed by torrential monsoons throughout Pakistan in July and August of the same year. Not only did people die as a direct result of the extreme temperature, but the severe heat led to cholera outbreaks in localized settlements around the largest economic hub, Karachi. Adding to the catastrophic effects of monsoon rain–related flooding was the effect of glacial melting that caused widespread damage to the country's infrastructure and contributed to loss of livelihood and loss of life.[2] In early January 2023, Reuters press reported that the result of heat stress, melting glaciers, and monsoon rains "killed at least 1,700 people, displaced around 8 million and destroyed key infrastructure."[3]

These extreme weather events were a direct effect of climate change and were not unique and infrequent occurrences but foreshadowed the events that demonstrate a pattern of climate related activities which continue to recur into the future. Recognizing that these events exact a financial cost on poor and marginalized countries that were once colonial outposts of developed countries and which hold very little responsibility for their current circumstances, the United Nations' Secretary General Antonio Guterres, in 2022–2023, led fund raising efforts explicitly on behalf of countries like Pakistan to secure financial reparations from developed countries like the USA, Canada, France, China, Saudi Arabia, and members of the European Union. In addition, the Secretary General sought funding from the Islamic Development Bank and the World Bank. The expectation to comply with the request for financial reparations related to "loss and damages" was simple. Many of the countries that will continue to bear the brunt of climate catastrophes, especially regarding loss of infrastructure, loss of livelihood, and loss of life, are most likely to have contributed the least to the problems exacerbated by decades of unbridled development. Understanding the importance of geographic area is essential to understanding the impact of climate change and the environmental conditions affecting human health. As noted previously, climate change is a relatively slow process – especially when one considers the age of the Earth. A common euphemism for slow progress is to move at a glacial pace because the creeping movement of glaciers was thought to be so slow. However, the melting of the continental glaciers, leading to increased sea level volumes, loss of biodiversity, and increased concentrations of atmospheric carbon dioxide, along with the recently recognized accelerated melting of arctic permafrost that is subsequently contributing to methane gas load in the atmosphere, is happening at a pace that has not been observed in the geologic record of the planet.

Recognizing and acknowledging the harmful effects of local and regional human activity on our environment is an important first step in identifying causal mechanisms for the rapidity of climate change. Moreover, it is important to acknowledge that these causal mechanisms can be changed only if we are truthful and admit that much of what we are doing in our quest to develop our civilizations is adverse to the existence of humanity. While we may continue to re-shape the planet, our unabated destruction of the biosphere will ultimately lead to the destruction of humanity, and although we will be gone, planet Earth, despite being scarred and battered, will continue to exist.

A simple example of the influence of human development, especially related to the built environment, was described by Kovats and Akhtari (2008) on the effect of urban centers as heat repositories. Heat repositories or heat storage locations result directly from structural designs of the physical infrastructure within the built environment. As human activities increase within the urban core, we often replace vegetation that once mitigated the heat-sequestering effects of concrete and asphalt with pavement and buildings. These activities can explicitly turn cities into "urban heat islands" that results in daytime storage of heat. The urban heat island releases heat slowly, which, in turn, leads to increased nighttime temperatures. Additionally, the development of urban heat islands can contribute to the intensity of rainfall, the formation of hail, and the severity of thunderstorms. The size of the urban area and the design of the built environment can have a measurable effect on local weather and, depending on proximity to coastal water and rivers, can contribute to the likelihood of flooding. In addition to the heat load from urban areas, cities become a major source for greenhouse gas emissions and thereby contribute to environmental impacts at a global level. The review by Kovats and Akhtari (2008) described projections of the Intergovernmental Panel on Climate Change (IPCC), which suggested that among the human health consequences attributed to climate change was the negative effect of extreme weather events on freshwater resources, which, in turn, will have a direct effect on food supplies.

Food security for animal and human populations depends on providing appropriate volumes of nutritional resources through agricultural processes and on the successful pollination of angiosperms (flowering plants). Flying insects, which include several types of bees, butterflies, moths, and even wasps, each contribute to the pollination of our plants and thereby have an essential role in sustainable agriculture and food production. Pollination is the primary stage in seed formation within plants (Wilcock and Neiland, 2002) and can be supported through a variety of animal species, which are primarily flying insects, but in some situations, wind pollination can support the transfer of pollen from the anther (male source of pollen) to the stigma (female receptor of pollen) among angiosperms. Pollinator colony loss and mass extinction of pollinators is a phenomenon that can be directly attributed to the activities of the Anthropocene and the results of climate change (Vieira et al., 2013). Human activity leading to loss of habitat, increased use of pesticides for land maintenance and/or enhanced agriculture production, and the emergence of undetected/unknown pathogens that target species of these insects are, in turn, causing the extinction of these essential constituents of the biosphere.

Both the bumble bee (*genus: Bombus*) and the honeybee (*genus: Apis mellifera*) are examples of essential insects that support continued sustainability of agriculture through the pollination of angiosperms within the entire biosphere. While it may seem improbable, it is entirely plausible that we could lose our bumble bees and honeybees in environments throughout the biosphere because of emerging infectious diseases (EIDs) such as deformed wing virus that specifically affects these creatures (Fürst et al., 2014). Losing pollinators through mass extinction as a result of human activity leading to climate change will be a causal mechanism in exacerbating food insecurity and negative human health consequences.

Human illnesses caused by malnutrition because of reductions in both the quality and security of food will increase in prevalence, as will the morbidity and mortality associated with vector-borne diseases like Zika, Lyme disease, West Nile virus, and malaria. These diseases were previously localized to specific geographic regions of the world, yet now, many are emerging in areas that were unscathed previously and are spreading at unprecedented rates. For example, while lyme disease was once thought to be localized to the Northeast region of the United States, originating from the town of Lyme, Connecticut, it is reported to be the most common form of vector-borne disease in North America (Ginsberg et al., 2021). Lyme disease is caused by the spirochete bacteria from the genus *Borrelia*.[4] The bacteria is carried by the black-legged tick (*Ixodes scapularis*) and passes on to humans when the individual is bitten by the tick. As Ginsberg and colleagues suggested, the spread of the disease may be dependent on the tick–host relationship and can involve more than one host. Having multiple hosts that can spread the disease increases the risk of infection to humans as well as the spread of the disease into areas that are frequented by any of the various hosts.

The effects of climate change on human health are not confined to the distant future. The effect of changing climates is happening, and we can both observe and measure the outcomes on human health. For example, Guirguis and coworkers (2013) reported that heat waves, resulting from extreme weather events and climate change, are linked directly to increased prevalence of heat-related illness. Seasonal mortality rate increases can be attributed to the increasing frequency, duration, and severity of heat-wave conditions in both urban and rural areas. Similarly, as heat waves increase, air quality decrease, and this relationship affects those with respiratory illness more severely, since many will have difficulty finding necessary relief from heat-related air quality degradation. Portier et al. (2010) referred to air quality because of the complex characteristics of atmospheric chemistry, which we know can increase risks for asthma and asthma-like symptoms, respiratory-related morbidity, and cardiovascular disease. Air quality is determined by the interactions of heat and humidity with the various concentrations of atmospheric elements. Predominantly, the air we breathe is made up of gases, with nitrogen contributing around 79% and oxygen contributing around 20%, while the remainder of gases include trace amounts of carbon monoxide, carbon dioxide, sulphur dioxide, and agricultural emissions like methane and ammonia (Kinney, 2018). However, add to the composition of air various types of molds, fungi, and airborne bacteria and viruses as well as particulate matter such as that which occurs with greater abundance in areas with wildfires. Combine all of these ingredients with the components of smog, which is especially prevalent in urban areas and is comprised of fog and smoke mixed with atmospheric gases, and we have the beginnings for an incredibly rich toxic soup for our breathing pleasure. In some countries, these effects are already sufficient to warrant air quality warnings for vulnerable individuals.

Although perhaps less intuitive than the physical health consequences of climate change, such as respiratory disease and nutrient deficiencies, the harms to mental health are every bit as real and as dire. An individual's identity is tied to their home and their surroundings. When we witness the loss of elements of our natural homes – be it through the erosion of land, urbanization of previously untouched habitats, destruction of natural landmarks, and so on – we may experience grief comparable to other forms of loss. Industries such as tourism, fisheries, and agriculture are vulnerable to climate change, too, with destruction of natural wonders (e.g., coral reefs, artic glaciers), alteration to water levels and reduced aquatic biodiversity, and increased risk of droughts and floods posing significant threats to the livelihoods and associated well-being of individuals and communities that depend on resource-based economies (Lemmen and Warren, 2004).

Additionally, climate change is affecting the mental health and well-being of populations as a function of its contributing role in natural disasters, such as floods, wildfires, and hurricanes, and the collective trauma that ensues from those crises. To disrupt the trauma and strife instigated by climate change, we need to examine the root causes of these intense weather calamities and pledge to move forward in a way that deals with existing damage without doing further harm to the biosphere. Again, given that climate change and related challenges are part of the wickedness of the problem, initiating a rapid-fire solution can easily become a cause of more severe future problems.

12.3 Planetary Health

Categorizing the impact of human activity on the health of the planet as the epoch of the Anthropocene helps us to situate current events within the geological time clock. However, recognizing the impact of this era on the interconnectivity of all life in the biosphere is of paramount importance to the sustainability of life on Earth. The term *planetary health* is based on an understanding of the interconnectedness of all living beings (Whitmee et al., 2015) and the acknowledgment that our sustained existence depends on a drastic human behavioral change across all aspects of life.

At every level of society, humans must realize and act on the threats that climate change presents to our existence.

> **The research evidence is clear. We are messing up the balance of life in the biosphere to a point from which we may never return.**

As the negative consequences of human impacts on the planet are becoming increasingly apparent, there is growing momentum to reverse our destabilizing influence on our environment. No longer can we ignore the loss of biodiversity among the constituents of the hierarchy that comprises the food chain, the continued disposal of particulate matter and toxic gases into the air that we breathe, or the wasteful exploitation of potable water resources. We have moved well beyond the ability to ignore our impact on the non-living/abiotic physical environment as our current exploitive actions perpetuate the cataclysmic degradation of the essential infrastructure that maintains the balance needed to sustain life on Earth.

For example, knowing the importance of sea ice as a naturally occurring solar radiation–reflecting mechanism should be enough to realize that without this "white shield" the Earth has no mechanism to reflect solar radiation. As we transition from our frozen tunic in the arctic and Antarctic regions to a fluid state through melting and calving of sea ice at the north and south poles, we increase solar heat absorption. Losing the ability to cool our oceans not only leads to a reduction in the ability of the oceans to absorb carbon dioxide from the atmosphere, but the increased environmental heat sequestration also changes the habitat on which billions of organisms depend.

Earth exists as a biosphere in which *Homo sapiens* are an integral part. Our existence as a species requires us to maintain the dynamic integration between the living and non-living components of the system that, together, act as a functional unit. Humans need to maintain the health of this ecosystem – to be the stewards of our planet – and maintain the positive state of all parts of the biosphere. We cannot overstate the importance that a healthy biosphere is fundamental to human health and hence to the sustainability of civilization. As Whitmee and colleagues reported, ecosystems within the biosphere provide multiple services, such as the availability of food and water, structural materials such as wood and fiber, and medicines and fuels. Ecosystems regulate life on the planet; they regulate climate, erosion, disease, and the replenishment of flora through continued pollination. Healthy ecosystems provide an aesthetic in which culture, recreation, and spirituality flourish.

Degrading or severely altering the biosphere within Earth's ecosystems not only impacts the individual constituent parts that comprise the ecosystems but will also lead to a direct negative impact on the health of humans. Degrade the ecosystem that enables global food production and observe increases in malnutrition and diseases associated with food insecurity. Degrade the ecosystem that ensures appropriate access to potable water and observe the increase in drought-related crop failures, dehydration, and pestilence associated with the lack of quality drinking water. Degrade the environment to the extent that it severely reduces pollinators and observe the starvation of millions of inhabitants across the biosphere.

Following his reading of the Intergovernmental Panel on Climate Change (IPCC) Working Group in 2021, UN Secretary-General António Guterres stated that our planet is in a code red situation regarding planetary health. As a first step to mitigate this code red situation, we need to increase awareness and understanding of planetary health. Next, we need to identify achievable actions so that every level of society can pursue meaningful and sustainable behavior change. For example, societies must begin the explicit departure from a dependency on fossil fuels and an expedient and efficient transition toward renewable energy sources. Communities must scale up programs that enhance carbon capture and storage through innovative mechanisms, a warning that has been supported by evidence of increased carbon load in the atmosphere[5] but largely ignored. As a society, we need to reduce consumption, reduce waste, and reduce unnecessary development of the environment, especially when such development is based on inappropriate policies and poor planning that lead to direct impact on the biosphere and biodiversity. Societies need to seek better ways to mitigate coastal erosion through the development of wetlands and salt marshes and continue to invest in the production of alternative energy sources such as wind, solar, and geothermal energy production.

Changing the behaviors of society by taking full advantage of a transformative utopian impulse for planetary health – that point at which society is inclined to take action that will transform society positively (Basso and Krpan, 2022) – is now more likely than ever before. Recent reports by the IPCC suggest that human activity got us into this mess, and so human activity can get us out of it. Our challenge is to spread the word, translate the knowledge, and continue developing strategies that eliminate the degradation of the biosphere.

12.4 Infectious Diseases

The COVID-19 pandemic provided the necessary impetus to advance the conversation on planetary health and the ways in which humans have disrupted the natural systems of life on Earth. The transmission of emerging infectious diseases (EIDs), many of which arise through zoonosis – the transmission of pathogens from animal to human (Jones et al., 2008, Han et al., 2015) – is well studied as a plausible vector of transmission for human contagion. According to Han et al. (2015), more than 1 billion illnesses are attributed to zoonotic infections worldwide each year. The emergence of the COVID-19 global pandemic is one such zoonotic infection that was not without forewarning (Jones et al., 2008). Research by Jones and coworkers included a review of some 335 EIDs identified between 1940 and 2004. The researchers found that the presence of EIDs was not a function of random occurrence but could be linked directly to increases in population density and population growth. Moreover, Jones and coworkers reported that EIDs were linked not only to zoonosis in a general sense, as may be anticipated with domesticated animals, but directly to unconventional pathogens arising from wildlife. In their comprehensive review, the authors reported that while more than 60% of EIDs were associated with zoonosis, more than 71% of these zoonotic-type EIDs were associated with pathogens from wildlife, specifically listing Nipah virus and SARS 1.

The work of Jones et al. in 2008 was extremely important to public awareness of global pandemic risk because it was the first analytical support for the suggestion that the "threat of EIDs to global health was increasing, 990." Likewise, noting that more than half of the zoonotic pathogens could be linked to wildlife, the authors explicitly stated that identifying the factors that increase contact between wildlife and humans is essential to developing predictive approaches to identify disease emergence and establishing strategies to prevent localized outbreaks and widespread contagion.

Later research by O'Callaghan-Gordo and Antó (2020) supported the presence of a transmission route for wildlife to human zoonosis by noting that the cause of the COVID-19 pandemic was attributed directly to open-air markets in Wuhan, China, where some 120 animals of 75 different species were sold. This plausible pathway for disease transmission was also affirmed in a separate investigation by the WHO, which reported its findings in February 2021.[6] According to O'Callaghan-Gordo and Antó, some of the animals sold at the Wuhan open-air market were alive and included puppies of wolves, salamanders, crocodiles, scorpions, rats, squirrels, foxes, civets, and turtles, all of which could be considered active vectors for transmission of emerging infectious diseases. However, the most important overlooked issue related to the transmission of pathogens from wildlife to humans is that the risk of producing a virus like COVID-19 (aka SARS-CoV-2) was predictable given the environment and what we had learned previously from the events which led to SARS I in Guangdong Province, China, more than 17 years earlier. In the earlier development of SARS I, it was believed that live bats were exposed to civets (a catlike mammal) which created an optimal pathway for disease progression between animal species. As O'Callaghan-Gordo and Antó suggested, despite having knowledge of routes for disease transmission and alerts from scientists that the current environment of live meat markets (not only in Wuhan but throughout China) was primed for another outbreak of widespread zoonotic infection, the authorities chose not to act (O'Callaghan-Gordo and Antó, 2020).

12.5 Conclusion

Without question, climate change is a real and present danger for humanity. As we have heard so often at all levels of society, ***climate change is a threat to our very existence***. The relationship between climate change and human health is demonstrated continuously by both direct and indirect effects on our morbidity and mortality. The pace at which climate change is occurring is not monotonic but is accelerating at a rate unprecedented in the chronological record of the planet. Now is the time to recognize and act on the direct and indirect effects of climate change on the specific health outcomes that include chronic diseases (e.g., cardiovascular and respiratory), injuries and fatalities from severe weather events (e.g., floods, landslides, heat waves, ice storms), emerging infections and vector-borne diseases (e.g., malaria, Zika, COVID-19, West Nile virus), mental health outcomes (e.g., stress, grief, and financial hardship resulting from disasters to the natural environment), and food insecurity and loss of freshwater resources, to name but a few of the observable and measurable outcomes. The negative consequences of planetary health and climate change are not only affecting the existence of humans but are also having a negative effect on all of our neighbours in the biosphere.

12.5.1 Discussion Questions

1   Considering that our planet has continuously evolved since it first emerged from the big bang, why should we be concerned with climate change now?
2   How is climate change associated with health and well-being?

Notes

1 The Australian Academy of Science. www.science.org.au/learning/general-audience/science-climate-change/1-what-is-climate-change retrieved February 10, 2021.
2 From "www.aninews.in/" July 10, 2022, retrieved January 9, 2023. URL: Searing heatwaves, torrential rains impact thousands in Pakistan (aninews.in).
3 From Reuters Press January 9, 2023, URL: Donors exceed Pakistan goal with pledge of more than $9 bln for flood recovery | Reuters.
4 From https://lymeguide.info/borrelia-bacteria/ retrieved on February 14, 2021.
5 Retrieved from Climate Change: Atmospheric Carbon Dioxide | NOAA Climate.gov Written by Rebecca Lindsey. Reviewed by Ed Dlugokencky. Published June 23, 2022. Accessed on July 5, 2022.
6 Retrieved February 10, 2021 www.cnbc.com/2021/02/09/who-outlines-wuhan-findings-on-origins-of-covid-pandemic.html.

References

Basso F, Krpan D. Measuring the transformative utopian impulse for planetary health in the age of the Anthropocene: A multi-study scale development and validation. *Lancet Planet Health*. 2022;6:e230–e242.

Chan M. Statement: (2008), *The impact of climate change on human health.* WHO. Creative Commons Licence: CC BY-NC-SA 3.0. Retrieved September 26, 2024, from https://www.who.int/news/item/07-04-2008-the-impact-of-climate-change-on-human-health#:~:text

Cianconi P, Betrò S, Janiri L. The impact of climate change on mental health: A systematic descriptive review. *Front Psychiat*. 2020;11. doi:10.3389/fpsyt.2020.00074

Folke C, Jansson A, Rockström J, et al. Reconnecting to the biosphere. *Ambio*. 2011;40(7):719–738. doi:10.1007/s13280-011-0184-y

Fürst MA, McMahon DP, Osborne JL, Paxton RJ, Brown MJ. Disease associations between honeybees and bumblebees as a threat to wild pollinators. *Nature*. 2014;506(7488):364–366. doi:10.1038/nature12977

Ginsberg HS, Hickling GJ, Burke RL, et al. Why Lyme disease is common in the northern US, but rare in the south: The roles of host choice, host-seeking behavior, and tick density. *PLoS Biol*. 2021;19(1):e3001066.

Guirguis K, Gershunov A, Tardy A, Basu R. The impact of recent heat waves on human health in California. *J Appl Meteor Climatol*. 2013. doi:10.1175/JAMC-D-13-0130.1

Han BA, Schmidt JP, Bowden SE, Drake JM. Rodent reservoirs of future zoonotic diseases. *Proc Natl Acad Sci U S A*. 2015;112(22):7039–7044. doi:10.1073/pnas.1501598112

Ireland V, Rapaport B, Omnirova A, Addressing wicked problems in a range of project types. Procedia Computer Science *Complex Adapt Syst. Publication 2* 2012. Conference Organized by Missouri University of Science and Technology, Washington DC; 2012.

Jones KE, Patel NG, Levy MA, et al. Global trends in emerging infectious diseases. *Nature*. 2008;451(7181):990–993. doi:10.1038/nature06536

Kinney P. Interactions of climate change, air pollution, and human health. *Curr Envir Health Rpt*. 2018;5:179–186.

Kovats S, Akhtar R. Climate, climate change and human health in Asian cities. *Environ Urban*. 2008;20:165–175.

Lemmen DS, Warren FJ, editors. *Climate change impacts and adaptation: A Canadian perspective*. Natural Resources Canada; 2004:174 p.

May RM. Why should we be concerned about loss of biodiversity. *C R Biol*. 2011;334(5–6):346–350. doi:10.1016/j.crvi.2010.12.002

O'Callaghan-Gordo C, Antó JM. COVID-19: The disease of the Anthropocene. *Environ Res*. 2020;187:109683. doi:10.1016/j.envres.2020.109683

Portier CJ, Thigpen Tart K, Carter SR, et al. *A human health perspective on climate change: A report outlining the research needs on the human health effects of climate change*. Environmental Health Perspectives/National Institute of Environmental Health Sciences; 2010. doi:10.1289/ehp.1002272 Available: www.niehs.nih.gov/climatereport

Robinson PN. Deep phenotyping for precision medicine. *Hum Mutat*. 2012;33:777–780. doi:10.1002/humu.22080

Sciberras E, Fernando JW. Climate change-related worry among Australian adolescents: An eight-year longitudinal study. *Child Adolesc Ment Health*. 2022;27:22–29. doi:10.1111/camh.12521

Steffan W, Crutzen PJ, McNeill JR. The Anthropocene: Are humans now overwhelming the great forces of nature? *Ambio*. 2007;36(8):614.

UCAR.edu. Layers of earth's atmosphere | Center for Science Education. https://scied.ucar.edu/learning-zone/atmosphere/layers-earths-atmosphere (accessed January 11, 2023).

Vieira MC, Cianciaruso MV, Almeida-Neto M. Plant-pollinator coextinctions and the loss of plant functional and phylogenetic diversity. *PLoS One*. 2013;8(11):e81242. doi:10.1371/journal.pone.0081242

Whitmee S, Haines A, Beyer C, et al. Safeguarding human health in the Anthropocene Epoch: Report of the Rockefeller Foundation – Lancet Commission on planetary health. *Lancet.* 2015;386(1007):1973–2028.

Wilcock C, Neiland R. Pollination failure in plants: Why it happens and when it matters. *Trends Plant Sci.* 2002;7(6):270–277. doi:10.1016/s1360-1385(02)02258-6

Index

Note: Page numbers in *italics* indicate figures, and page numbers in **bold** indicate tables in the text